AF782823

TOP DOCS

Managing the Search for Physician Leaders

Second Edition

by George F. Longshore

American College of Physician Executives
Suite 200
4890 West Kennedy Boulevard
Tampa, Florida 33609
813/287-2000

Copyright 1999 by Longshore + Simmons. All rights reserved. Reproduction or translation of this work beyond that permitted by applicable copyright law without the permission of the author is prohibited. Requests for permission to reprint or for further information should be directed to the Permissions Editor, ACPE, Two Urban Centre, Suite 200, 4890 West Kennedy Boulevard, Tampa, Florida 33609.

ISBN: 0-924674-71-7
Library of Congress Card Number: 99-62337

Printed in the United States of America by Hillsborough Printing Company, Tampa, Florida.

About the Author

George F. Longshore is President of Longshore + Simmons, Conshohocken, Pennnsylvania. The firm, previously called Fulton, Longshore and Associates, Inc., has been providing executive search; physician recruitment; and organization, compensation, governance, and market-related consulting services since 1979. Mr. Longshore has a bachelor of arts degree and has pursued a master's degree in business administration from Temple University, Philadelphia, Pennsylvania. He has held executive positions with two investor-owned hospital management corporations and was director of human resources for several divisions and subsidiaries of Ford Motor Company. Mr. Longshore has appeared before local and national audiences of management professionals, addressing such topics as succession planning, the evolving role of the hospital executive, executive recruitment, and physician compensation. He has served on the board of a Pennsylvania hospital and is currently a trustee of a Washington, D.C., institution of graduate education. Mr. Longshore is a Certified Healthcare Consultant (CHC).

Acknowledgments

No work of this magnitude could have been accomplished without the active support and encouragement of many persons. Longshore + Simmons' professional staff provided critical review and advice in the early stages of the book's development. Clients provided not only fertile ground for the many examples used throughout, but also the push needed to continue the manuscript development during those inevitable lulls. In particular, we are indebted to our friends at Abington Memorial Hospital, Abington, Pennsylvania; AtlantiCare Health System, Atlantic City, New Jersey; Anthem Blue Cross and Blue Shield, Cincinnati, Ohio; Hackensack University Medical Center, Hackensack, New Jersey; University of Pennsylvania Health System, Philadelphia, Pennsylvania; and Temple University Medical School, Philadelphia, Pennsylvania; for their help and advice.

A very special thanks to Linda Brown, without whose organizational abilities through many rewrites I would have been hopelessly lost.

Dedication

To my wife, Joanne, who put her life's dreams and career goals on hold so that I could take a risk. Her love, support, and advice over the past 20 years are as much a part of this book as the words on paper.

To my children, Alicia and Janelle, who laugh at my jokes, respect my advice, and whose love allows me to be fulfilled as a father. I am forever proud of you both.

To my "spiritual director" Reverend William A. Guerin, OSFS, whose prodding, encouragement, and always-present support has allowed me to achieve what I could not alone. Father "G" showed me, by his example, how to live in the present moment.

Preface

I stared at the cover of the first edition of *Top Docs* with a considerable amount of skepticism. After all, I had been involved in a number of physician searches, chairing some, and should know what to look for and how to look for it. The rubric was well known: appoint a committee, select a chair, change the committee, place advertisements, talk to colleagues, review lists of candidates, interview some, extend an offer, enjoy the result.

But it didn't always go swimmingly. The process took too long. Expectations by the committee members were not always well defined or synchronous, although most agreed that all acceptable candidates should walk on water. The nature of the interviews was defined by previous experience rather than by the specific requirements of the position. From the eyes of the candidate, attributes of the position and institution could be enshrouded in an impenetrable fog. Evaluations by the candidates' colleagues never seemed less than laudatory. The negotiation process could be difficult and even contentious. The individual selected might be more tolerated than enjoyed, and might not have the critical skills demanded by the position.

Given the rapid changes in the world of medicine, would skills that served leaders well in an earlier time be appropriate today? It was time to rethink both the process and its objectives. Perhaps *Top Docs* was worth a look. After all, we physicians were trained to recognize our limitations and to seek consultation when necessary. Should our behaviors as physician administrators be any different? Curiosity and apparent need overcame skepticism. *Top Docs* beckoned more insistently. From its first warning, "Take Care to Get What You Like," the book presents a systematic, knowledgeable, and perceptive series of chapters detailing the responsibilities of both institution and candidate so that each arrives at a mutually satisfactory choice. The book concludes with a series of appendices offering helpful data, approaches, and forms of use for a wide variety of searches.

Top Docs II both expands and refines the information from its predecessor. A new Part I, "Deciding to Search," outlines necessary preliminary steps that must be taken before the search committee, now described in Part II, is appointed. The role of a search consultant is described, and must come to the attention of even those in academia as an increasingly important force in helping select the right candidate. Part III adds a chapter on the department review process, a useful step that defines the department (or other administrative unit) as it now exists and establishes a vision for its future development. Parts IV and V, dealing with the candidates, negotiation, and compensation, are now defined by subheadings that more clearly identify content areas. As a whole, the Table of Contents, with its listing of Parts, Chapters, and subheadings, provides a quick overview and review of the search process.

Those of you who are involved with any dimension of the search process will both enjoy and benefit from this monograph. It systematizes what can become a very disjointed process. It provides a clear track for those new to the search process and a wealth of information and necessary reminders to all.

Richard J. Kozera, MD
Executive Dean
Temple University School of Medicine
Philadelphia, Pennsylvania

Foreword

"Take Care to Get What You Like...."

If more search committees kept George Bernard Shaw in mind, this book might not be needed. "Take care to get what you like," admonished the acerbic playwright and essayist, "or you will be forced to like what you get." Far too many health care organizations currently lack the will, the savvy, and/or the resources to take proper care in finding and hiring the key physician-leaders on whom their very survival may rely.

Today is no time to "be forced to like what you get" in a physician leader who will head up a major clinical product line that produces revenue for a hospital; a vice president of medical management who will help the health system implement and manage "risk"; or the medical director who will be responsible for effectively and creatively managing the utilization of the MCO's network. Pressures on U.S. health care institutions and organizations continue to proliferate. The coming years promise new twists on the already-daunting problems of competition, shrinking reimbursement, external oversight, rapidly expanding and expensive technology, and the demands of an aging population. Additional regulatory, economic, societal, clinical, and ethical issues are bound to emerge. Without visionary leadership, a health care organization's prospects for prosperity are dim.

Medical leaders both in health systems and in managed care organizations must be more than just the "clinical presence" and must become key members of the executive team devising innovative, creative solutions to business problems.

As the shifting health care scene draws them into decision-making beyond the boundaries of traditional medicine, physician leaders—chiefs of medicine, surgery, geriatrics, oncology, neonatology, etc.—must be more than clinicians. Finding these multifaceted and forward-thinking individuals has become an increasingly complicated process. Many organizations continue to tackle it the old-fashioned way. Sometimes that works. But more and more often, traditional recruitment and search committee procedures founder on the shoals of contemporary reality. Unplanned physician leadership selection has brought grief to more than one hospital, health care system, or MCO in the past. In the future, poor choices are bound to pose more profound hazards.

Misdirected efforts to recruit department chairs and other physician leaders—the "*Top Docs*" of a variety of institutions across the country—may be launched by well-meaning, but disorganized, search committees. Or they may be the outcome of searches mounted by poorly composed, divided committees whose internal relationships rival those of Shakespearean drama. In these cases, the very important purpose of these committees gets snarled in the process of the search. Eventually, only outside assistance can tease apart the tangled strands of the endeavor.

There are ways to avoid the pain of the physician leader recruitment and search committee process. This book stands as a guide to planning and managing a successful search for key physician leaders. To those who initiate, chair, or serve on physician leader search committees, it offers a systematic and strategic approach to defining, seeking out, evaluating, and selecting viable candidates in a timely fashion. It emphasizes closure—something that commonly eludes medical search committees in their attempts to win commitment from the "*Top Docs*" they want. Designed as a user-friendly manual, the book takes committee chairs and members, as well as anyone engaged in the recruitment process, step-by-step through the search process and provides documents and checklists that will support their efforts.

Leaders who have been appointed to a search committee, and those engaged individually in the physician leader recruitment process, will benefit most directly from this information. In the long run, their organizations will also benefit from it, of course. Health care systems' chief executive officers and academic deans, along with hospital trustees/board members and senior executives in health care human resources, finance, and physician liaison roles, will also find useful material in the following pages. Physicians who wish to expand their roles to include executive responsibilities and residents who are considering a physician executive career path will learn of the credentials, skills, personal attributes, and philosophies that characterize the best candidates for top physician-leadership jobs. Overall, this book tells how to "take care to get what you like." It offers guidance and insight into the organization and direction of a process, and a cast of characters, that have too often gone ill-defined and unmanaged.

The new edition of *Top Docs* incorporates observations regarding the acute need for qualified, capable, and talented physician leaders in today's integrated health care delivery systems, the necessity of partnering between physician leaders and the strategic decision makers in health care organizations of all types, and the need for these organizations to recruit the "best of the best" physician leaders for survival in the new millennium in health care.

Compensation data and expense projections have been brought current; forms and other useful tools have been refined and improved. A new section on departmental review and its application as a tool for search committees has been added, and an explanation of the search committee process in academic settings has been strengthened in recognition of the rapidly rising demands placed on physician leaders in academic roles.

I hope you enjoy the results.

George F. Longshore
President
Longshore + Simmons
Conshohocken, Pennnsylvania.
July 1999

Contents

APPENDICES

Part I

Deciding to Search (The Preliminaries)

CHAPTER 1

Determining the Organizational Need

At some time in the life of every organization, there is the need to search for leadership. This may come at the creation of the organization, during its growth and maturity cycle, or on the downturn. Wherever the organization is in its life cycle, it is important for it to step back and to fully assess the conditions generating the need for new leadership. Without the benefit of a well-defined strategic plan, an organization can make a critical mistake in the appointment of leadership in various roles throughout the organization.

Regardless of how mature or immature the organization is, one consistent emotion precedes the search for all key leadership roles—the organization first "feels the need" for leadership. As an organization is just being formed, the need for leadership is more apparent than at any other time. It is obvious to the person or persons who put the endeavor together; someone needs to lead it. However, during the growth cycle of the organization, there are times when intuition is a better guide to leadership appointment than a predetermined plan. Pressures on the organization that is not getting things done, is not accomplishing its goals, is slipping financially, and is losing market share will begin to focus on creation of the new leadership position after everything else has been tried and the organization is stressed and frustrated with lack of progress.

The CEO of a managed care organization in a mid-western state was frustrated with his business units' poor showing in quality surveys reflecting community opinion of the service. While the financial results were okay, as were other business indicators, the organization was not gaining market share. The chief medical officer, while well respected in the community, lacked sufficient managed care experience to significantly change the behavior of the physicians in the network. In spite of servicing 300,000 covered lives, the organization employed only a chief medical officer and a part-time medical director. After more closely studying what each of these physicians was actually doing day-to-day and comparing their performance to what was expected, it was apparent that both were stretched too thin and that the appointment of at least one and possibly two additional medical directors was warranted to not only fuel but also sustain the growth of this managed care organization.

A vacancy can occur in an existing leadership position that makes the decision to search for a replacement easier. However, even in this situation, the organization should look closely at the requirements of the position—not only today but into the future—and at what is expected of this role before seeking candidates. The candidate that you place in the position today may not be appropriate for the same position in a year or so.

A major university-affiliated health system had embarked on an aggressive program of practice acquisition and on development of a strong well-regarded physician network. At the head of this organization was a chief medical officer who, once the system acquired more than 125 physicians, was finding it difficult to aggressively pursue and value additional physician practices to allow the organization to get to its goal of 400 primary care physicians. A search for an associate medical director was begun, with the primary focus of assisting in targeting and valuation of new physician practices. It should have been obvious to the organization that, although it was undergoing organizational stress at the time, it would soon accomplish its goal of acquiring 400 physician practices and the associate medical director role would either shift in a dramatic way or no longer be required. This would create either redundancy in the organization or turnover when the services of the associate medical director were no longer required.

Good thinking, therefore, is required before actively seeking a physician for a leadership role in the organization. Focusing on the strategic plan and direction of the organization will help ensure appropriate timing and scope of the position.

A national managed care organization, in attempting to manage its transition from an indemnity business to a pure managed care business, was faced with the challenge of "ramping up" its medical services organization. Under the indemnity model, few if any medical directors with significant responsibilities were in place (figure 1, page 5). Under the "managed care" model, physicians in key leadership roles throughout the organization (both corporate and divisional) would be needed to change behavior of physicians in the participating network. After soliciting key executives throughout the organization for their input and insights, several medical services organizational models were presented. All of these models provided for changing the organizational structure as the business matured.

The model chosen (figure 2, page 6) incorporates a "group practice model" concept. The newly appointed medical directors will, at least initially (6-12 months), be viewed as a "group" of medical directors sharing responsibility for a wide range of organizational, operational, and programmatic issues as this newly emerging managed care organization gets on its feet. The medical directors will be available as needed throughout the organization to "triage" problems as they occur. After 12 months, a more defined role for each medical director, aligned either geographically or along product lines, is expected to occur. Candidates identified for the interim roles need to be appropriate for longer term organizational needs.

Before embarking on the search for a physician executive, an organization must be certain that the identified need is consistent with the organization's strategic plan and that the position is not being created to mask the deficiencies of others in the organization or of the organization itself.

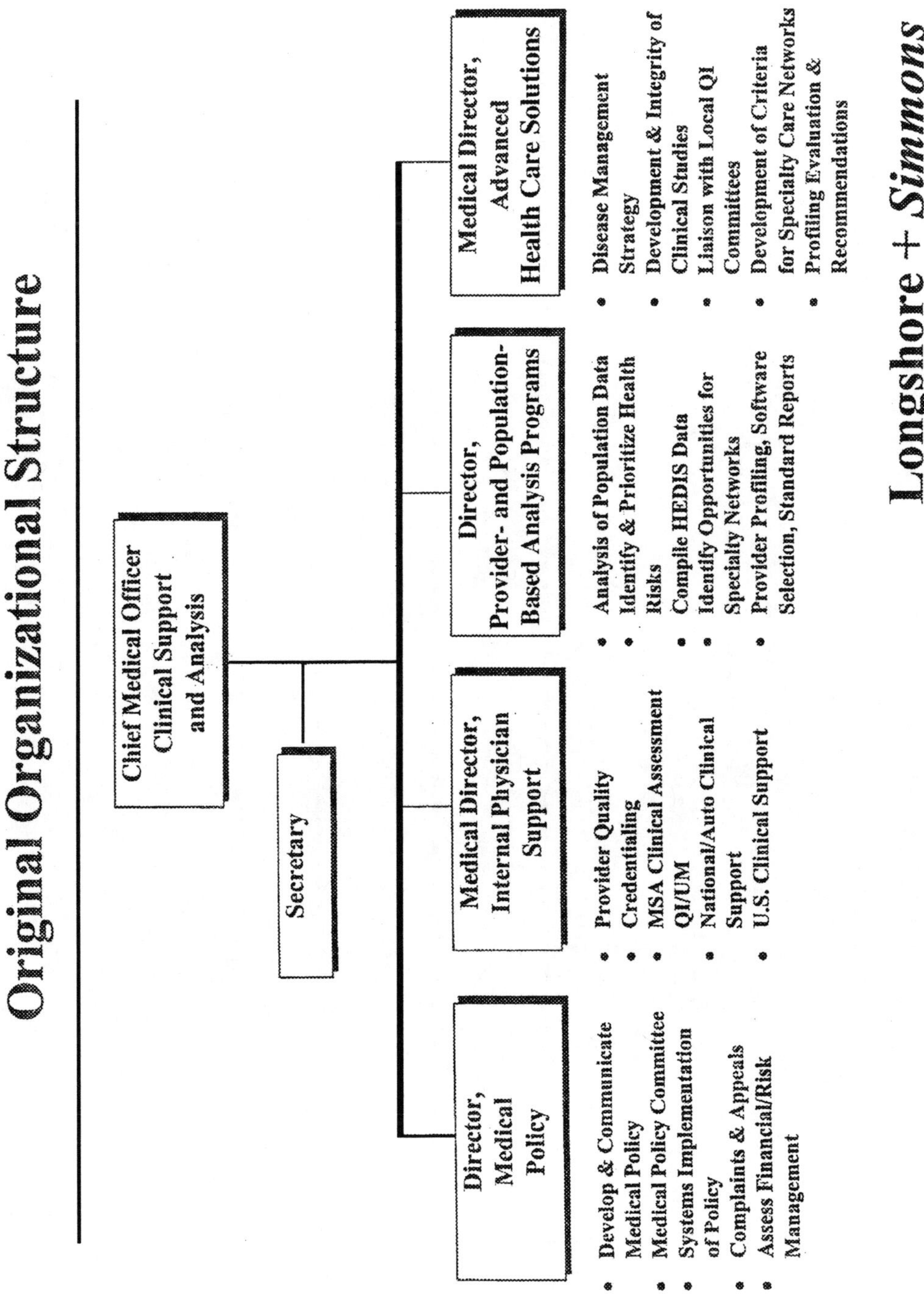
Original Organizational Structure
Chief Medical Officer
Clinical Support
and Analysis
Secretary
Director,
Medical
Policy
• Develop & Communicate
Medical Policy
• Medical Policy Committee
• Systems Implementation
of Policy
• Complaints & Appeals
• Assess Financial/Risk
Management
Medical Director,
Internal Physician
Support
• Provider Quality
• Credentialing
• MSA Clinical Assessment
QI/UM
• National/Auto Clinical
Support
• U.S. Clinical Support
Director,
Provider- and Population-
Based Analysis Programs
• Analysis of Population Data
• Identify & Prioritize Health
Risks
• Compile HEDIS Data
• Identify Opportunities for
Specialty Networks
• Provider Profiling, Software
Selection, Standard Reports
Medical Director,
Advanced
Health Care Solutions
• Disease Management
Strategy
• Development & Integrity of
Clinical Studies
• Liaison with Local QI
Committees
• Development of Criteria
for Specialty Care Networks
• Profiling Evaluation &
Recommendations
Longshore + Simmons

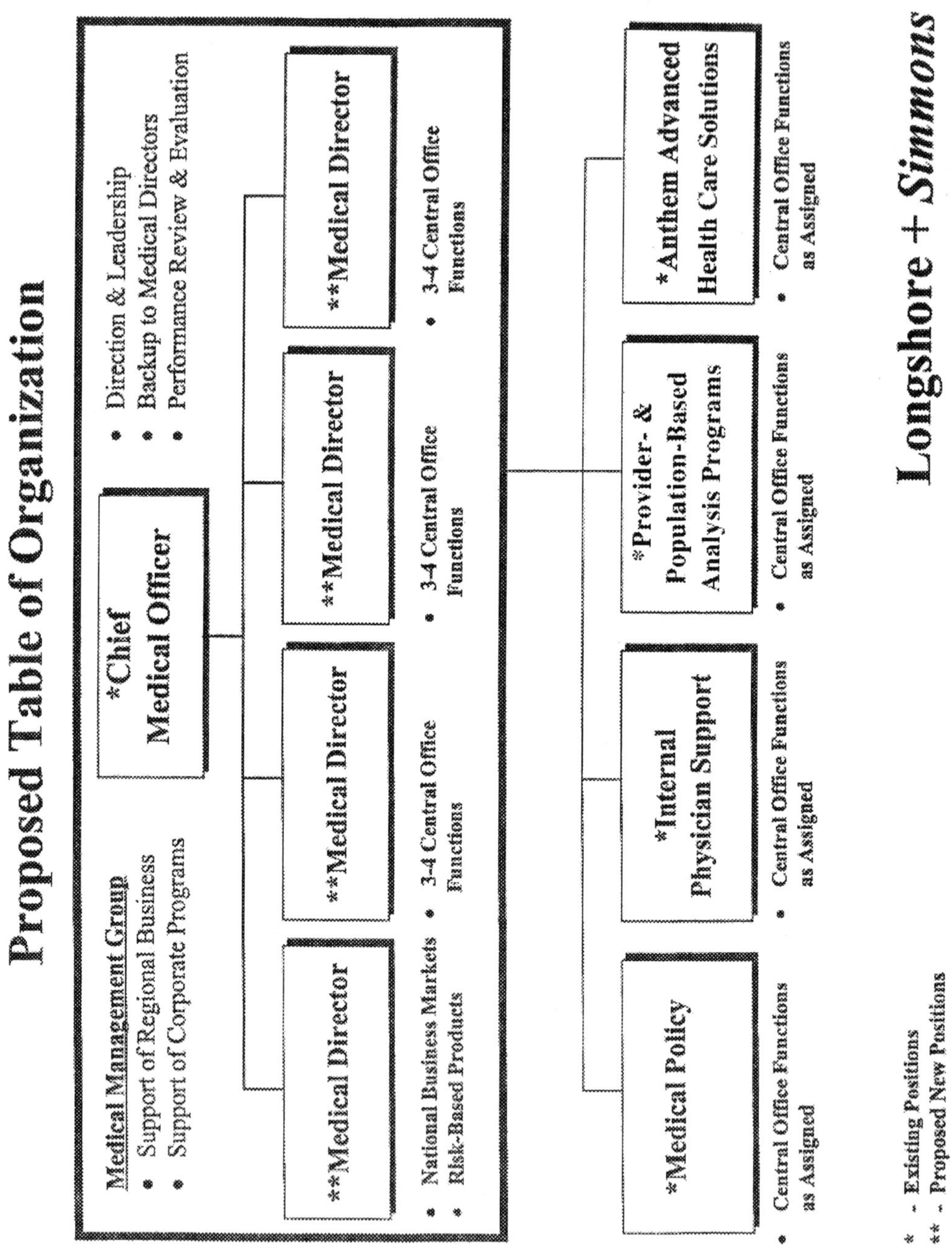

Proposed Table of Organization
Medical Management Group
• Support of Regional Business
• Support of Corporate Programs
*Chief Medical Officer
• Direction & Leadership
• Backup to Medical Directors
• Performance Review & Evaluation
**Medical Director
• National Business Markets
• Risk-Based Products
**Medical Director
• 3-4 Central Office Functions
**Medical Director
• 3-4 Central Office Functions
**Medical Director
• 3-4 Central Office Functions
*Medical Policy
• Central Office Functions as Assigned
*Internal Physician Support
• Central Office Functions as Assigned
*Provider- & Population-Based Analysis Programs
• Central Office Functions as Assigned
*Anthem Advanced Health Care Solutions
• Central Office Functions as Assigned
* - Existing Positions
** - Proposed New Positions
Longshore + Simmons

CHAPTER 2

Defining the Position

The "Position Specification"

The most important, and frequently the most overlooked, step in any recruitment effort is development of the position specification or the job description. If you do not know what you are looking for, it will be impossible to find it. If recruiting a physician to a leadership position is like putting together a jigsaw puzzle, the position specification is the frame of the puzzle. The frame gives the puzzle its shape and limits and is used to define results.

Any recruiting effort, whether alone or with outside assistance, that does not have a well-developed position specification is likely to founder. The position specification, if properly developed, will be used throughout recruitment activity to measure candidates and to ensure adherence to predetermined position requirements. It will prevent the organization from "straying" too far from its objective.

Engaging the Organization

It is a wise leader who seeks the insights and the opinions of others in the organization before attempting to define a key physician-leadership position in his or her organization. Engaging others in the organization who are above, below, and around the position for which you are recruiting will not only provide good practical suggestions that help define the position, but also allow members of the organization to feel part of the recruitment process.

For instance, in the recruitment of a senior vice president for medical affairs, the CEO of a health system sought comment from trustees, executive staff, medical staff leadership, and voluntary physicians. This was accomplished through individual interviews that were conducted "in confidence." It is always a good idea to involve the "customers" of the position for which you are recruiting. These comments can then be assessed and incorporated in the position specification. Copies of the position specification should be shared with all who provided comment.

Developing the Position Specification

A well-developed position specification for any position includes the following major sections:

- **The Organization**—A description of the organization with enough detail to allow prospective candidates to quickly assess the scope of the employer organization and to allow the organization to "market" itself to prospective candidates.

- **The Need**—Why is the position open; what circumstances created the opportunity? For instance, retirement, resignation, or re-assignment of the incumbent; organizational growth; merger; affiliation; new lines of business?

- **The Opportunity**—A description of the major responsibilities and accountabilities of the position.

- **Qualifications**—What minimum education and experience requirements an individual needs to possess in order to become a candidate.

- **Compensation and Benefits**—What base compensation, total compensation, benefits, and perquisites are attached to the position.

The following position specification was developed for a community teaching hospital needing a vice president for medical management:

Position Specification

Title: Vice President, Medical Management

Client: St. Agnes Medical Center
Philadelphia, Pennsylvania

St. Agnes Medical Center is a well-regarded, 236-bed acute care Catholic teaching hospital and a member of the 13-hospital Franciscan Health Care System. Having served the Philadelphia metropolitan community for more than 100 years, the Medical Center provides high-quality patient care in a compassionate environment that emphasizes community service. The medical staff encompasses over 250 active members. Recognized services include an outstanding regional burn center and a freestanding hemodialysis unit. The emergency department handles approximately 18,000 visits per year. The facility also serves as a training site for osteopathic interns and offers training in general practice, internal medicine, and general surgery. Allopathic residents from four area programs also rotate through the burn center.

The Opportunity:

The Medical Center seeks a committed physician whose experience and vision will provide effective leadership for the institution. The Vice President of Medical Management will have the opportunity to assist in strengthening existing clinical programs and in identifying new program needs. He or she will also assist the Medical Center and the medical staff in continuing to develop a strong managed care orientation.

Reporting administratively to the President and Chief Operating Officer, the Vice President of Medical Management will be responsible for overall medical/ administrative affairs related to health care delivery and medical staff management of patient care. He or she will work closely with the President of the Medical Staff and the Medical Executive Committee and all Department Chairs in administering medical staff affairs and in achieving the strategic goals of the Medical Center.

Responsibilities:

Medical Staff Affairs

Function as a member of the regional senior management team as a patient, physician, and clinical care advocate. Ensure proper functioning of medical staff affairs by working cooperatively with the President of the Medical Staff, Clinical Chairs, and appropriate medical staff committees to:

- Develop annual goals and objectives with the medical staff executive committee—coordinate objectives of the medical staff with overall institutional objectives.

- Oversee compliance with the bylaws and rules and regulations of the medical staff and keep them current and competitive.

- Counsel medical staff on the administrative applications of cost containment, risk management, quality assurance, and utilization review—ensure that administration and the governing body fully appreciate the implications of medical staff decisions regarding professional activities.

- Assist in development of the medical staff, including recruitment and supervision of house staff.

- Ensure proper credentialing and reappointment processes, and evaluate and enhance delineation of privileges for medical and allied professional staff.

Medical Center Affairs

As a member of the medical center's management team, participate in systemwide planning and management processes and assist in determining operational goals to meet current and future patient care needs. Work closely with the President/COO and the President of the Medical Staff to:

- Provide leadership to medical and management staff in the areas of clinical consolidation, clinical information system development, clinical integration, clinical outcomes development, managed care development, and medical management and medical staff affairs.

- Provide educational, consultative, and technical assistance in managed care—including contracting, health care delivery and financing mechanisms, integrated delivery system development, insurance, and physician/hospital relationship development. Support development of a coordinated managed care infrastructure—including a primary care network, contractual relationships, and participatory activities for the medical staff.

- Support identification, development, and refinement of physician support services and programs—including practice acquisition, primary care network development, physician office management, and physician recruitment.

- Comply with medical requirements of JCAHO and other licensing/regulatory or accrediting bodies. Ensure that the Medical Center operates through policies and practices consistent with the philosophy and values of the Franciscan Health System.

- Direct and lead collaborative relationships with member boards, medical center management teams, medical staffs and other partners, and the Sisters of St. Francis of Philadelphia to ensure effective communications and clinical operational effectiveness.

- Provide public relations services on medical matters. Represent the medical center at appropriate meetings in the Catholic health care community and in other health care organizations.

Qualifications:

The successful candidate will demonstrate leadership ability and qualities that reflect a thorough understanding of the needs and concerns of private practitioners as well as a solid working knowledge of Medical Center operations. Experience and personal traits should allow the candidate to build and maintain effective relations and credibility with the medical staff, Medical Center administration, the Board of Directors, and lay/health professional communities. The Vice President of Medical Management should embrace and live the core values of the Sisters of St. Francis of Philadelphia and the operational philosophy of the Franciscan Health System. Additional qualifications include:

- Board-certified physician with at least 10 years' clinical practice experience and five years within a medical administrative role with a large health care organization. Advanced degree in business or health care preferred.

- Significant administrative and/or staff experience in hospital medical affairs, including general affairs, department management, medical staff leadership, case management, physician development, and managed care.

- Results-oriented individual with a proven track record of accomplishment in clinical consolidation, clinical integration, clinical outcome development, medical staff/hospital partnering, managed care development, and strategic partnering.

- Leadership style that engages participation and respect of medical administrative staff and results in win/win outcomes. Employs a participative, collaborative management style and is an effective team builder.

- Personal traits of maturity, fair mindedness, consensus building, and diplomacy. Supportive of and committed to the mission and values of a Catholic hospital.

The following position specification was developed for a corporate medical director in a large, managed care organization.

Position Specification

Client: Health Partners
Philadelphia, Pennsylvania

Title: Senior Vice President for Medical Affairs/Medical Director

Reports To: President/CEO

Company Overview:

Health Partners is the only not-for-profit, provider-sponsored HMO in the Philadelphia region. Owned by leading teaching and community hospitals, Health Partners was one of the first health plans to develop a model that involves shared financial risk between the HMO and contracting providers. One of its chief assets is its global sub-capitation contracts with all its major provider entities.

With more than 120,000 members and $238 million in annual revenue, Health Partners is the third largest HMO in the Philadelphia area. It is a major contractor under HealthChoices, the Commonwealth of Pennsylvania's mandatory managed care program for Medicaid recipients. This program expands Health Partners' relationship with Pennsylvania's Department of Public Welfare (DPW), which began in 1985 when DPW endorsed creation of Health Partners under a national program funded by the Robert Wood Johnson Foundation and cosponsored by the Health Care Financing Administration (HCFA) and the National Governors' Association.

In 1995, Health Partners entered into an administrative services agreement with a hospital consortium to provide Medicaid managed care services in Lehigh and Northampton counties. This venture, known as Partnership Health Plan (PHP), uses Health Partners' existing infrastructure for administrative support while transferring risk down to PHP for the management of medical services. Since its inception, PHP has consistently met growth targets and is now the largest plan of its type in the region, with nearly 7,000 enrollees.

In 1996, Health Partners was one of a highly select group of applicants chosen by HCFA to be a contractor under Medicare Choices, a three-year Medicare demonstration program. The contract with HCFA became effective February 1, 1997, with the first enrollees on May 1.

Health Partners also offers a commercial product, although it has traditionally limited enrollment in this line of business to its own employees. After 12 years of operations, enrollment across all Health Partners' product lines is as follows:

Program	Enrollment
Medicaid	113,114
Partnership Health Plan	6,843
Medicare	1,110
Commercial	273
Total	121,340

Although the so-called 75/25 requirement for commercial enrollment was recently eliminated by Congress, Health Partners previously obtained a congressional waiver of this requirement. This waiver, granted to only a handful of plans nationwide, is indicative of the Plan's well-regarded reputation and political support. Health Partners has a waiver of the 50/50 Medicare requirement under the HealthChoices program.

Health Partners' service area currently covers Philadelphia, Bucks, Montgomery, Delaware, Chester, Lehigh and Northampton Counties. Health Partners' Medicaid product is offered in all of the above areas to individuals eligible for Medical Assistance. The commercial service area includes the counties of Philadelphia and Delaware and southern portions of Bucks and Montgomery Counties. Health Partners' Medicare product, however, is currently limited to Philadelphia County.

Health Partners is owned by seven of the Philadelphia area's most prominent university and community teaching hospitals. These institutions and their affiliated networks make up the core of Health Partners' delivery system:

- Allegheny University Hospitals
- Temple University Hospital
- St. Christopher's Hospital for Children
- Hospital of the University of Pennsylvania
- Albert Einstein Medical Center
- Episcopal Hospital
- Frankford Hospital

Health Partners' total network includes more than 44 hospitals in its seven-county service area. In addition, Health Partners has contracted with more than 1,025 primary care physicians and 3,400 specialists. More than 80 percent of the Health Partners physician network is board-certified. Health Partners subcontracts for certain medical and ancillary services, including vision, dental, behavioral health, laboratory, and pharmacy.

Health Partners performs all core administrative and operational functions internally. An IBM mainframe-based proprietary information system processes claims and enrollment and feeds a data warehouse. Adjunctive to this system are applications for credentialing, quality assurance, and decision support. Technology enhancement is ongoing, with acquisition of imaging/OCR capability and expansion of an EDI interface.

Revenues for all product lines in 1997 are projected to be $238 million, a 19 percent increase over 1996 levels. Medicaid currently accounts for 98 percent of all revenue, although this percentage will fall as Medicare enrollment increases over the next three years. Broad risk-based contracting, innovative medical management, and lean administrative overhead has enabled Health Partners to generate net surpluses in 10 of the past 12 years.

The Position:

The Senior Vice President for Medical Affairs (SVPMA) is responsible for all medical aspects of Health Partners, with particular focus on effectiveness and efficiency of the health care delivery system. As an integral member of the executive management team, the SVPMA serves as an officer of the Board of Directors and reports directly to the President and Chief Executive Officer.

The SVPMA provides leadership and guidance to credentialed providers and their professional staffs, with the goal of maintaining the highest level of quality in health care delivery. In addition, the SVPMA is responsible for managing medical costs and for working with the Chief Operating Officer, the Chief Financial Officer, the Chief Information Officer, and other directors and managers to build a provider network that supports and nurtures Health Partners' goals.

Specific responsibilities include, but are not limited to:

- Developing and recommending annual utilization benchmarks and quality improvement strategies.
- Establishing annual budget and work plan for Medical Affairs Department.
- Managing delivery of medical services through globally sub-capitated integrated health systems to achieve corporate goals for medical cost management and quality improvement.
- Managing delivery of medical services in a manner that is consistent with NCQA standards for accreditation and with state and federal regulations and program requirements.

- Participating in the strategic planning process as it relates to risk arrangements, provider incentives and responsibilities, and use of technology to promote efficiencies and communications.
- Overseeing Medical Affairs Department's implementation of corporate and departmental goals.
- Integrating the operations of Medical Affairs Department with all other key areas of the organization.
- Overseeing staff support for successful operations of the Medical Affairs Committee and its subsidiary committees.
- Reporting on Medical Affairs Department's plans, goals, and activities at Board of Directors meetings.
- Providing medical leadership to internal constituencies (i.e., Board, staff).
- Representing Health Partners to external constituencies, including the Department of Public Welfare and the Department of Health, as well as the provider community and other managed care organizations.

Qualifications:

- Board certification, preferably in a primary care specialty or in preventive medicine.
- Ability to balance service provision with cost containment, evidenced by three to five years' experience in a managed care organization.
- Demonstrated leadership skills in a team environment and a commitment to high-quality care.
- Prior experience managing physicians in a business environment.
- Exceptional interpersonal, problem-solving, and communication skills. Maturity and experience to lead a growing health care organization.
- Complete working knowledge of business and financial principles related to prepaid health care practice. Medical Assistance and/or Medicare risk experience is highly desirable.
- Ability to establish oneself as a clear, decisive leader in a rapidly changing environment.
- Personal style that conveys confidence and enthusiasm and engenders trust in others.

Compensation:

Health Partners offers a competitive base salary and a comprehensive benefits package, with relocation assistance as appropriate.

In addition to defining the organization and why the need exists for the position, a well-developed position specification will allow a prospective candidate to see the scope of responsibilities attached to the position and the qualifications required. This will provide candidates with the opportunity to properly assess themselves against the qualifications of the position and decide whether it is something they would like to pursue.

The qualification section is the template that the employer organization will use to measure prospective candidates. This section of the position specification is the most important and the most necessary. It is in failing to properly define the qualifications of prospective candidates that most organizations fumble recruitment. This section will be referred to continually throughout the course of the search and before major decisions are made regarding selected candidates. If the organization is being forced by market conditions or other pressures to consider candidates who do not meet the qualifications, serious discussions are warranted. Either the qualifications section of the position spec needs to change, or the organization needs to redouble its efforts to locate candidates with the original set of qualifications. (See Part IV, Chapter 16, for more on the position specification).

Compensation

There are many different opinions about how specific you should be in stating the compensation range, the benefits, and the perquisites for an executive position. One preference is to be as general as possible so as not to turn off prospective candidates who see the cash compensation as too restrictive. "Don't turn them off before you get them in the door." (See Part V for more on compensation.)

Gaining Approval of the "Spec"

Whether the step is required or not, those who provided input to the development of the position specification should be given a copy of the final specification. This is especially important when working with search committees for physician leadership positions. All members of the committee will have provided their input to this document, and they need to review it one last time before it is approved and put into the market.

Chapter 3

The Work Plan

A work plan is an organization's road map to effectively recruiting a physician-leader. Whether working with or without a search committee, every organization should develop a work plan outlining each of the major steps in the recruiting process and the timing of each step. This will give all involved a better idea of the task at hand and realistic goals for its completion.

The major steps in any search process are:

- Information Gathering
- Position Specification (Developing and Approving)
- Targeting a Pool of Candidates
- Screening Candidates
- Interviewing and Evaluating Candidates
- Reference and Credential Checking
- Closing the Employment Offer

Each of these steps can be easily defined with estimated times for accomplishment and assignment of responsibilities. Appendix 1 shows a work plan constructed for the recruitment of a Chair of Obstetrics and Gynecology

Laying out a work plan in advance lets everyone know what is going to happen when and who is responsible for it. This document will generally go a long way to keeping the process on track and to controlling the anxieties of organizational members as appropriate work unfolds.

The first three or four steps of the work plan are very predictable and easier to adhere to than are the latter steps. The latter part of the process can drag on and be distorted if scheduling of candidates is not aggressively undertaken and managed. Vacations, holidays, and other travel restrictions can add months to a search that is not well defined in advance. (See Part III, Chapter 14, for more on the work plan.)

CHAPTER 4

The Pool of Candidates

Defining the Pool

Strategizing regarding identification of an appropriate pool of candidates frequently requires outside assistance. The health care field abounds with professional and trade organizations and newly erupting special interest groups and organizations, and it is very difficult to keep up with these developments. For instance, the *Directory of Associations* lists more than 150 organizations that represent physicians. Some of the organizations typically targeted for physician executive candidates include:

- American College of Physician Executives
- Society for Physicians in Administration (Medical Group Management Association)
- National Association of Managed Care Physicians
- American Medical Directors Association (long-term care)

The first step in development of any strategy for appropriately attacking the market for candidates is to think about where those candidates currently reside (in what types of organizations and in what settings) and how you would attract their attention. For instance, if you are searching for a vice president for medical affairs for a community teaching hospital, you might attempt to identify physicians who are currently holding similar titles in smaller institutions. The American College of Physician Executives could be a resource in this regard. Those physicians could be reached by advertising in *Physician Executive magazine* more quickly than by newspaper or other trade journal advertising.

Physicians who are interested in utilization management/quality management are likely to be members of the American Board of Quality and Utilization Review Physicians (certifying organization) and the American College of Medical Quality (formerly American College of Utilization Review Physicians). These physicians could be attracted by advertising in the *American College of Medical Quality Focus, Diplomate Focus Newsletter, and the Journal of the American College of Medical Quality* or by mailing to them directly.

Accessing the Pool

By and large, the most effective way of attracting candidates from a pre-defined pool is through direct personal contact. The search industry has thrived because of the effectiveness of direct solicitation of prospective candidates for positions in other organizations—in other words, "pirating" individuals away from other organizations through a direct personal selling technique. If an outside resource, such as a search firm, is used to attract physicians to leadership roles in an organization, this is most likely the approach that will be used. Individual organizations are reluctant to directly solicit candidates from competitors. They are more likely to entertain those candidates if they come forward on their own or through a third party. Advertising, while expensive, has not proved to be very effective in recruitment of physicians to senior leadership positions. The reasons for this are varied:

- Physicians belong to a variety of organizations, and, to be effective, advertising needs to be finely targeted to the pool.

- Senior-level executives are reluctant to respond to ads because of their concern about the confidentiality of such inquiries.

- It takes time and effort to respond to an ad. Many successful physician executives are not in the market and are not prepared to take these steps.

Direct mail campaigns, whether by the organization or by a professional recruiting organization, are not effective unless they are followed up quickly with phone calls. The response rate of a direct mail campaign jumps from 2 percent to more than 15 percent with direct telephone follow-ups.

The Internet is increasingly becoming an effective tool for organizations and professional recruiters alike. Specialized medical and health care services' web sites, such as those listed below, allow better targeting of prospective candidate pools when an opportunity is listed on these web sites. Physicians interested in executive positions and/or in making a move to new positions, will increasingly be using these web sites for job prospecting. The Internet offers ease of response and quick response time to the interested candidate. The dangers, however, for the candidate are similar to those encountered in responding to newspaper advertising. One of the dangers of listing an opportunity on the Internet is that the whole world becomes aware of the opportunity. Therefore, much as with newspaper and journal advertising, you can become quickly inundated with responses from prospective "candidates."

- www.acpe.org (American College of Physician Executives): Job listings; resume bank; resume composition help.

- www.namcp.com (National Association of Managed Care Physicians): Job listings.

- www.nejm.org (*New England Journal of Medicine*): Extensive job listings, including chair/chief/director category.

- www.ama-assn.org (American Medical Association): Links to *JAMA* and other specialty publications with job listings.

- www.acphysci.com (Academic Physician & Scientist): Job listings, including an administration category with various subcategories, from medical director to dean positions.

- www.physemp.com (Physicians Employment): Job listings for all specialties, including physician executive and director categories.

Handling the Responses

Once candidates begin responding to your opportunity, each needs to be handled in a professional manner. Timely responses, whether letters of *no interest* or signals of *serious interest*, need to be handled within a week to 10 days of receipt. More than one organization has found itself on the receiving end of blistering criticism, both directly and in the media, regarding lack of response to submitted resumes or curriculum vitae. A routine clerical activity can be set up at the beginning of the recruitment activity to ensure that the task does not get overwhelming and that appropriate records are kept.

CHAPTER 5

Searching Alone or Assisted?

Experience shows that it takes from six to 12 months to complete a physician-leader search. Medical staff search committees working on their own can take from 12 to 24 months. The assistance of an experienced executive search consultant will reduce the average time spent to four to six months. The sooner the consultant becomes familiar with the organization's needs and involved in the search committee's formation and procedure, the shorter the search is apt to be.

How do you know whether you really need a search consultant? The fact is, some organizations do quite nicely on their own, accomplishing their physician-leader searches in short order. The key to their success is inevitably a highly focused chair assisted by an equally clear-sighted, small search committee, all sharing an unflagging dedication to the same goals. Certain that it has achieved such a combination, a search committee can proceed independently without qualm. Or, as the following case history demonstrates, it can meld its own strengths with those of a search consultant to leap tall orders at a single bound.

The secret of a super-search committee is to leap in unison under strong, proactive leadership. Cedars Hospital, a 447-bed community hospital in a northeastern city of some 50,000 people, accomplished this, filling a critical position in just 90 days. The search committee's mission: to replace the hospital's departed open-heart surgeon and two associate surgeons quickly, so that the entire open-heart program could resume activity.

Michael B. Anthony, President of Cedars, explained that the cardiac surgery program was the hospital's advertising leader, the "hype of the hospital," so that the search was vitally important to the institution. The time without an open-heart leader would be costly; Cedars did not want to be out of the open-heart market for long. Moreover, it had a full-blown cath lab in place, "but until we had an open-heart surgeon again, we couldn't do complicated caths. And we had decided not to reduce staff in the cardiology program while the search was going on. Even though that put the expense side of our income statement out of line, we thought it was prudent. If we had laid people off, in our opinion it would have taken significantly longer to bring the whole program back up again once the new chief came on board."

A sense of urgency is not uncommon in top doc searches, but whether it contributes to committee confusion or committee cohesiveness has to do with how it is harnessed. At Cedars, the hospital's president was the catalyst and, for three months, gave 60 percent of his time to orchestrating and implementing the search for a cardiac surgeon.

The committee he assembled consisted of seven members, including the president of the medical staff and himself. All were carefully chosen from disciplines that would interact with the open-heart surgeon (they included cardiologists, surgeons, and an anesthesiologist) to form a balanced group. No single specialty would have undue influence. A very senior surgeon—an obstetrician/gynecologist—was named chair. There were political considerations in choosing the committee members. "At Cedars, thoracic and vascular surgeons can't do open-heart surgery, and the open-heart surgeon can't do thoracic or vascular procedures. It's a political hot potato. One large surgical group wants an open staff instead, but the board and administration didn't and don't. The open-heart surgery program had only been up and going for two-and-a-half years when this search began, and maintaining its quality required monitoring and controlling in a closed program." The hospital thus sought to sign an open-heart surgeon to an exclusive contract.

Anthony had no difficulty in choosing search committee participants in collaboration with the president of the medical staff. The board elected not to have a representative sit on the committee, because it saw itself as a policy-making body that had decided to engage the new surgeons and viewed the medical staff as the body that would execute that policy.

The committee met and immediately developed a position specification. There was no disagreement on these criteria. With time of the essence, Anthony and the group then decided to take some unconventional routes toward the goal, not waiting for one step to be done before taking another and eschewing the traditional method of "sending letters to potential candidates, waiting for CVs, reviewing all the CVs, and sending letters of interest back." They also identified certain steps that a good outside consultant could take more efficiently than they could.

As soon as the position spec was agreed upon, Anthony engaged a search consultant, gave him the spec, and asked him to start the search at once. An unexpected benefit—but one that Anthony recommends other search committees plan for in advance—was that the consultant had been successful in recruiting cardiac surgeons. "The quicker you can get to a search consultant with a track record, the quicker your search will go."

The search consultant was hired primarily to identify candidates and make early contact with them. It was his job to describe the available position and the candidate criteria to these prospects; to tell them about the search committee, the hospital, and the "culture" (of which he got a sense by attending one of the search committee's first meetings); to inform them of the exclusive contract arrangement required; to gauge their level of genuine interest; and to eliminate any who could not or would not meet these needs. Anthony acted as the consultant's liaison with the search committee during this candidate identification process, which was characterized by fast and furious phoning and faxing among hospital, consultant, and candidates. Each day, Anthony informally shared all incoming information with the search committee chair and the president of the medical staff.

In keeping with the unconventional approach, Anthony worked during this same period to activate his own "old boy network," contacting people who he knew might provide candidate leads. His request was, "Is there anyone in your program ready to be a chief and willing to bring some associates along?" His efforts yielded a number of CVs. This procedure risked overlap with the search consultant's efforts—something that could have caused conflict over fees. Defusing that possibility at the outset, Anthony came to an understanding with the search firm: Only CVs that the consultant generated on his own or that inadvertently duplicated those generated by Anthony (of which, in the end, there were none) would be counted in determining the search firm's final fee.

After two and a half weeks, 12 suitable candidates had been identified—about half each by Anthony and the consultant. Here, the consultant bowed out, and the search committee proceeded on its own to evaluate the surgeons' qualifications. Using a ranking technique, it assessed each CV according to the candidate's fit with the spec, his or her (yes, "old boy network" notwithstanding, one candidate was a woman) experience in community hospital and private practice settings (versus university and academic medicine settings, for example), and other relevant criteria. The committee winnowed the candidate list to five. Anthony called each of them directly "to find out if they were really serious about a new position or just shopping" and to make sure that truly interested candidates would be available to begin in October 1990, because timing was critical.

Anthony and the search committee had a few more ideas to help speed the recruitment process along. "We required each of these five candidates to bring their wives when they were interviewed. We wanted to be sure the final candidate and his wife liked our community. We didn't want to take the chance that a spouse arriving late in the hiring process would veto the city and change a prime candidate's mind about accepting the position." Not content to wait until candidates were free to visit, Anthony and other search committee members took to the road themselves.

"To keep things moving, it was faster to arrange for some of our candidates to talk with us in their locations than to schedule a two-day trip to ours. A candidate from Houston agreed to meet us halfway, so the search committee chair and I went to see him in Denver. Also, the two of us, along with a cardiologist, drove to the home of another candidate and talked with him there for four hours. The chief financial officer went with me to Dayton, Ohio, to interview another candidate, and we went to Atlanta to see yet another." On each trip, the Cedars representatives carried with them copies of pro formas; draft contract outlines; the compensation and benefits package being offered; and clear descriptions of the three-year, exclusive, guaranteed arrangement with practice plan and noncompete provisions. This ensured that the candidates had a solid understanding of the terms of potential employment.

All this jet-setting took place within a four-week period. Between trips, the recruiting team reported the interview findings and candidates' status to the committee, and the candidates and their spouses began to arrive at Cedars for on-site visits and interviews with other committee members. At the same time, Anthony was back on the telephone, referencing the five candidates in traditional and not-so-traditional ways, including calling the heads of nursing at their current hospitals and at institutions where they had previously worked "to find out how they worked with nurses and other people. Did they upset nurses? How did they treat the cath lab techs?" What these professionals thought was as important as what the candidates' peers thought about their management and interpersonal skills. Anthony also checked on candidates' external relations by talking with community organizations in areas where the candidates worked. "If one belonged to the Rotary, I called the president of the local Rotary and asked, 'How does this person get along with people? How are his speaking skills etc.?'"

Finally, three candidates—surgeons from Pennsylvania; Dayton, Ohio; and UCLA—were left in the running, all of them acceptable to the medical staff. After open discussion, the search committee declared its role in the process to be finished. The members' position was that they should judge candidates only on their clinical credentials and capabilities, their interpersonal skills, and their fit with the spec, leaving hospital administration to tend to contractual matters and to close the deal. So Anthony again took to the air.

Now he is amazed at his juggling act, having negotiated contracts with all three candidates simultaneously. By choice, no attorney accompanied him; at this juncture, Anthony didn't want confrontation (or bills). He believed that the incoming physician and the hospital CEO would inevitably meet and that the moment should come sooner rather than later. "Naturally, there are going to be some sticking points, but the idea was to find out who would come to terms with a business deal we could both live with and then bring in the attorneys for the fine print." About 50 days into the 90-day period, this was just what happened when Anthony closed a deal with the choicest candidate, from UCLA. Final contract negotiations consisted mainly of lawyers and clients completing documents. Because the candidate was well aware of the hospital's business parameters—had, in fact, agreed to them in principle—this stage took only two-and-a-half weeks.

The contract itself was modeled after that of the departed open-heart surgeon and associates, plus more than two years of experience with revenues and billing for the program. The hospital had been billing for the program through one of its subsidiaries, providing a good idea of the income that could be generated for the professional component. The search committee knew what the disposable income level of a cardiac surgeon should be as a result of nationwide salary data it had collected, and it knew that Cedars' numbers were competitive. It supplied information to candidates about the local cost of living, such as geographical comparisons of utility bills.

The new open-heart surgery program leader brought just one other surgeon with him to Cedars, leaving a vacancy on the staff. The original search committee decided not to mount a search for that cardiologist; it determined that, once the new chief was on board, it was up to him to hire another associate, as in any other private practice. Soon after arriving, the new chief did so, using his own "old boy network."

Time was plainly a great motivator in Cedars' search. Intensely concentrated on getting the open-heart surgery service up and running again, the search committee took some extraordinary measures that proved both appropriate and cost-effective. A routine search could have taken substantially longer, and the hospital would have lost the revenues from cardiac patient care during that time, while still maintaining the full cardiac team (except surgeons). Anthony acknowledges that spending 60 percent of his own time on the search "may have been unique to my commitment. At the beginning, I gave myself that window of time to concentrate my efforts, because the open-heart surgery program was so important to me. I don't know that hospital CEOs would routinely get on as many airplanes as I did and negotiate contracts."

Nevertheless, Anthony advises other hospitals to take a similar approach to recruiting physicians to lead programs that are highly significant to their institutions. CEOs who balk at devoting such a large chunk of their time to the search might involve a search firm more heavily to speed the process, he concedes, but adds, "It takes a CEO's involvement to get it done. If you allow things to linger along, they'll linger along. If you want to bring them to a conclusion, my experience has been that it works best for the physician and the CEO to sit down alone in a room and work out the deal, get it down on paper, pretty much shake hands on it, and then give it to the lawyers or whomever to put in their protective language." Asked if most physician-leaders in today's litigious climate are willing to do this, he replied, "By all means!"

Internal Resources

In earlier chapters, the roles and uses of executive search consultants in the search committee process have been explored. There are still other players who may come from beyond the committee's ranks, or from outside the organization entirely, to take part in the recruitment and hiring of a new physician-leader.

One who may seem a likely participant in the process usually is not. Although many hospitals now employ them on their administrative staffs, *in-house recruiters* do not, as a rule, work with search committees looking for physician-leaders. In-house recruiters are quite busy recruiting and negotiating with community-based and/or employed network physicians (family practitioners, obstetrician/gynecologists, orthopedic surgeons, for example) and, in some cases, with new physicians for the hospital-based medical staff (e.g., anesthesiologists, pathologists, emergency medicine specialists). Of necessity, their point of view is normally task-oriented, rather than broad-based and long-range. They would be hard-pressed to commit the substantial amount of time needed to produce and process candidates for a key leadership position.

Few internal recruiters have developed a network of the sort of top docs who would be the appropriate candidates for such a position. Nor do they customarily have the requisite clout to steer a possibly argumentative search committee in directions that (whether individual members like it or not) reflect the health care organization's larger goals. Unpleasant exchanges may dot the search committee process, and it takes a seasoned professional to keep them from draining members' resolve and interest. In addition, it is seldom a good career move for an in-house recruiter to be the bearer of bad news to the high-level physicians charged with hiring a new clinical leader; yet, that is a role that someone must play in the search committee process.

On the other hand, even the crabbiest search committee member will at least listen to what an experienced outside search consultant has to say, if only because of the way it is said. A consultant is skilled at igniting fires under search committees in order to shed light on the entire committee process. The combination of heat and light is often just what members need to rouse themselves from addled torpor or bristly indignation. It follows that they can then proceed more quickly and forthrightly toward the committee's real goals.

Attorneys for the hospital and the candidate will become involved in the recruitment process. For the health care organization, the legal issues that impinge on the hiring of a physician-leader need to be considered before the committee sits down to work. And it is the board of trustees/directors and/or the organization's CEO that must decide on and articulate those issues in accord with the organization's overall physician-leadership strategy.

Among the matters warranting discussion are the form that a contractual relationship with the about-to-be-sought physician-leader will take (e.g., fee-for-service, salaried, some combination?); the duration of the contract; whether or not the new physician-leader will be permitted to maintain a clinical practice; whether to mandate termination of the physician's medical privileges, without recourse to the grievance procedure available under medical staff bylaws, upon termination of the contract; and whether to require that the candidate attain or keep board certification, as well as full medical staff privileges at the hospital, in order to retain his or her position. These seemingly mundane items can present major problems in closing a search if they have not been considered and resolved at the outset and if they are not clearly communicated to the search committee members and to each candidate.

Involvement by attorneys in the course of a search—whether they represent the institution or a candidate—can be obstructive. It is hard enough to keep a search committee's proceedings simple and to the point. Attorneys can be truly helpful at the very beginning of the process (in developing a framework) and at its end (in constructing the final contract with the chosen candidate). In between, they are usually superfluous (although they are not likely to see it that way). Even the letter of intent that is ordinarily sent to the preferred candidate need not involve lawyers, as Michael Anthony at Cedars Hospital demonstrated. After conversations with the candidate, it can be put together by the committee chair and the hospital CEO, as long as the agreed-upon framework is honored.

Attorneys who are not familiar with physician contracts and with the legal issues inherent in the physician-hospital relationship have often stood in the way of closure of a physician-leader search. Many prime candidates have been lost to hospitals, and many ideal opportunities have been lost to candidates, through the use of unpracticed attorneys. Beware the candidate who brings a brother-in-law to contract negotiations!

Selecting and Working with a Search Consultant

The circumstances and leadership of Cedars' open-heart surgeon search do not always come together when a top doc position needs to be filled. Sometimes a search committee has worked on its own for months or even years before the chair or hospital CEO acknowledges that the unthickening plot needs a *deus ex machina*. Whatever the reason for calling in a search firm, its first job will be to develop and exhibit a thorough understanding of the situation and a rapport with the search committee members. Until this is done, the firm's credibility is limited, and so is its ability to comb the market for candidates who fit all the hospital's needs.

For these, among other, reasons, a search firm that specializes in recruiting physicians and other leaders for health care organizations offers the best value. Although "physician recruitment" firms have proliferated in recent years, the vast majority of them focus their skills on recruiting hospital staff, community-based, and HMO physicians often directly out of residency programs—not on searching for top docs.

An executive search firm with broad health care expertise, on the other hand, will draw on a large national or international network of contacts among experienced senior physicians in all specialty areas. It is accustomed to dedicating its time, energy, expertise, and resources to closing deals with such physicians. It will have independently studied a variety of marketplace issues that should be factored into a search committee's work. It will be savvy about the psychology, as well as the economics and politics, of job change among physicians at or nearing the peak of their careers. It will be ready to use this knowledge in structuring a customized package for the chosen candidate. And it will be intimately familiar with the search committee process.

Search committee members do not, as a rule, engage frequently in recruitment activities such as interviewing and negotiating. They are thus well-served by the support of a search consultant when it comes to the myriad rules and obligations that dog the employment process. A thorough and up-to-date knowledge of regulations that affect how a physician can practice and be compensated is absolutely necessary. So is expertise in the ticklish "isms" (sexism, ageism, racism, ethnocentrism, etc.) that abound in today's hiring environment; there is seldom a human resources specialist attached to a search committee to provide guidance on these issues. Search committees may have valid, supportable reasons for turning away female, foreign-born/trained, or older candidates, but unless they present them correctly, they and their institutions are going to end up embarrassed (or worse).

Another legally precarious area for a hospital has to do with improper referencing of a candidate's background and prior performance. Well-intentioned but uninformed search committee members have all too often jeopardized a candidate's current employment by checking his or her background through the "old boy" network. In this day and age, such loose cannonading poses legal liabilities for institutions. An experienced search consultant can manage these and other issues representing potential exposure for the hospital.

Overall, a specialized physician-leader search consultant almost inevitably possesses better, more up-to-date knowledge of marketplace conditions than a search committee working alone. Such input does tend to enhance both the quality and the speed of the committee process.

In choosing an outside consultant, be aware that there are two types of "executive search" firms. A *retainer* firm will bill for services over the course of the project on a regular, predetermined schedule. A *contingency* firm will bill when a candidate is placed or accepts the client's offer. Usually among the latter are those that call themselves "physician recruitment" firms. They often approach physicians, seeking to work with them to find a practice opportunity. They operate as traditional employment agencies in this regard, and they usually bill on a contingency basis. Specialized executive search firms are asked by organizations to help top management and/or search committees locate and hire candidates for senior clinical or administrative leadership positions. They are paid on a retainer basis, which provides an economic incentive to perform well, since at least part of their fee is at risk until the assignment is completed.

Health care organizations generally use only one executive search firm per search, although it is possible that more than one firm may be involved in separate searches at the same time for the same hospital. Both individual hospitals and multihospital systems sometimes contract with firms for the recruitment of *all* their physicians. These are not exclusive contracts, however; the hospital or system has the right to use another firm for a search if it sees fit. The contracted firm usually does give the hospital a fee discount, however.

In order to make optimal use of the services of a search firm, organization executives and search committee members should keep in mind that the main reason for engaging the firm was to make the committee's job proceed more smoothly. Therefore, the organization should take every advantage of the "outside expert's" presence. Let him or her set deadlines, decision points, and interview schedules. It is the consultant's job to tug the organization and search committee members along at some points, to redirect them at others, and to restrain them at still others—all the while behaving like the soul of diplomacy.

Work with a consultant throughout the recruitment process as though he or she were your chief mediator. Whether interceding in intra-committee rivalries, administration-committee disputes, or candidate-committee encounters, a mediator shuttles between the parties involved. He or she is there to gain a wide perspective, understand all sides of an issue, communicate concerns, pose questions, and present the positions of one party to another. A consultant may, for instance, "prep" candidates for their meetings with various organizational representatives or search committee members: "Dr. Doe may seem a little negative. That's because he's worried about competition from you." Or, "Here's how Dr. Roe has approached other candidates she's interviewed." By taking this tack, rather than representing a single party, the mediator gains trust, respect, and a thorough comprehension of everyone's views.

These assets become particularly important in a physician-leader search once the to-ing and fro-ing are over and all parties have settled on a final candidate. The search consultant must then articulate the most reasonable positions of, and to, the organization and the candidate—the beginning of negotiations. The mediator role is then at its trickiest and most valuable stage.

Indeed, contractual closure can be extremely dicey without the help of a mediator. Often, one or both parties will be adamant about some negotiating items—usually ones related more to practice or organizational issues than to compensation. It is important to allow the search consultant to be the one who gets "dirty" as negotiations proceed and as tough issues are debated. The consultant is there to keep both search committee members and organization executives out of the direct line of fire, helping them to avoid confrontations that might sour relationships and lead to problems in the near and distant future. The same is true when closure nears; the consultant's job is to obviate the necessity for candidate and organization members to butt heads. Without a mediating influence, organizations and candidates frequently alienate each other in face-to-face arguments. Unfortunately, this usually happens just when the taste of closure is on both their tongues. Many a good candidate has been lost after such a run-in, especially when he or she is unaware of the organization's nonnegotiable positions.

For instance, a certain candidate for chief of physiatry in a 300-bed hospital in a suburban New Jersey community wanted the exclusive right to do electromyelograms (EMGs). In other settings, this would have been a perfectly reasonable request. But, at this particular hospital, members of the existing neurology staff had, over the years, built up quite a lucrative practice by doing all EMGs. Had the committee directly refused the candidate an exclusivity arrangement, he would have withdrawn. However, because the candidate had had the opportunity to explore the issue with the search consultant first, and the search consultant had been able to apprise the candidate of the EMG situation at the hospital, the prospective chief of physiatry was spared a direct declaration to an unreceptive committee. Instead, he was persuaded to delay his demand for immediate EMG exclusivity and to accept a phased-in approach—a period of years during which he could develop his own EMG practice with the support of the hospital. By diplomatically mediating this compromise, the consultant enabled the search committee to fulfill both its hiring and its assimilation support functions.

A search committee formed to locate a new chief of radiology did lose its best candidate because of inflexibility and the absence of a seasoned consultant. The committee inappropriately stuck to its guns in stating that the new chief be required to hire two existing staff radiologists; neither was board-certified, and one was no longer even board-eligible. The preferred candidate, not wanting to be saddled with "a less than qualified staff," broke off negotiations. On reconsideration, the committee decided that it was probably not a good idea to restrict a new chief. So, it approached its prime prospect again, offering to negotiate a "trial period" for the two existing staff radiologists. Too late. The best candidate was irrevocably lost, and the committee had learned that, if a deal is to close, someone respected by both sides must tactfully orchestrate compromises acceptable to each.

Actually, you should expect a consultant to work toward this goal throughout the search committee process, whittling down the number of items that are nonnegotiable on any side, for too many nonnegotiables normally mean "no deal." Just as market data are used to educate the committee about what is necessary to attract the best candidate, they can be used to secure a more reasonable position from the candidate. Items such as physician staffing per case, average CME time, expense allowance, and malpractice coverage costs are all arrows in the quiver of an experienced search consultant.

When it's time for the deft maneuvers of contract negotiations with the chosen candidate, the consultant (still keeping the parties apart) will first negotiate the easiest items, leaving the more troublesome ones for the final phase, when both candidate and committee are most eager to close. The objective is to end up with a "win-win" feeling for all parties. An "I win/You lose" attitude on either side might get the candidate, but it spells trouble for the future of the relationship.

TOP DOCS

Part II

The Search Committee

CHAPTER 6

Why Bother?

Perhaps it is some innate compulsion to bring new blood into the tribe, this search process. After all, our ancestors wandered the plains, not just hunting and gathering but occasionally raiding other groups, too. Taking prisoners who could expand the tribe's gene pool enhanced adaptability and the odds of survival in an unforgiving environment.

In health care organizations, the current version of this ancient quest for adaptability and survival takes place in a complex and demanding business environment. We no longer take prisoners, but we do seek to cross-fertilize abilities, accomplishments, and vision. Today, the ritual induction of new members into the "tribe," especially those deemed leaders, is incorporated in the activities of the search committee for medical leaders.

Is this an archaic practice? In this day and age of the ubiquitous consultant, when huge, generalized firms offer all things to all people and small firms sell arcane knowledge of the tiniest marketplace niches, one might question why a health care organization would continue to use search committees at all.

The reason has to do with the "tribal" nature of the health care profession. Physician candidates for leadership positions in hospitals are not selected purely on the basis of aptitude. They are also chosen for their "fit" into the "tribe"—that exclusive club of members of the medical staff of any hospital. Who can better determine "fit" than current club members? Hence, the medical staff search committee—still viable after all these years and, in increasing numbers, required by medical staff bylaws.

Sample By-Law Language: Protocol for Search Committees for Chairs and Chiefs of the Medical Staff.

8.8-1 Search Committee

a. *A vacancy in the position of Chair of a Department or Section Chief shall be announced at a regular business meeting of the Medical Staff. A Search Committee shall be appointed to fill such vacancies according to this Section 8.8-1.*

b. *Committee size should not be limited, and the Committee should be composed of at least two members of the Board of Managers, the President of the Hospital or his designee, and at least four members of the Medical Staff to include the President of the Staff or a designee. The Chair of the Board of Managers shall appoint the Board members, and such appointments should be approved by the Executive Committee of the Board of Managers. The President of the Medical Staff shall submit his/her recommended appointees to serve as the Medical Staff membership on a Search Committee for a Departmental Chair to the Executive Committee of the Medical Staff. The Executive Committee of the Medical Staff will, at the following Executive Committee Meeting, approve or alter such recommendation.*

c. *When practical and feasible, a member of the Department or Section in which a vacancy exists should be on the Search Committee as one of the four Medical Staff members. The departing Chair shall not have a vote on the Search Committee in regard to his successor, but may serve as an advisor to the Committee, if it so desires. If the vacancy is for a Chiefship, the Department member of the Search Committee shall be the Chair of the Department, and shall have veto power over any selection of a Chief in the Department; however, such a veto must be supported in writing, stating, in detail, the reasons why the Search Committee's recommendation is not acceptable.*

d. *The Search Committee shall elect its own Chair.*

e. *It shall be the responsibility of the Search Committee to explore in depth the past and present activities, from both a patient care and medical education point of view, of the Department or Section in which a vacancy for Chair or Chief shall exist. It shall also delineate present strengths and weaknesses within the Department or Section and estimate what future improvements and expansions might be anticipated.*

f. *At least a three-fourths affirmative vote of the Search Committee is necessary for the recommendation of a candidate for Chair or Chief to the Board of Managers.*

g. *If possible, the Search Committee should be convened at least one year before a vacancy for Chair or Chief exists.*

h. *Where a financial contractual relationship is necessary, the President of the Hospital and/or his designee shall meet with a candidate to conclude a satisfactory agreement.*

i. *In the event that the Search Committee is delayed in obtaining a satisfactory candidate, the incumbent Chair and/or Chief, or a person recommended by the Committee, can be appointed temporarily by the Board of Managers.*

The reality of health care provider organizations is that the board of directors/trustees cedes to the CEO the authority to hire a clinical leader. But that physician will be a tribal outcast until he or she attains medical staff privileges through the credentials committee of the medical staff. That isn't likely to happen unless the physician-leader has been accepted as a member of the club. Neither acceptance nor privileges would follow if a CEO hired a physician-leader without the active participation and support of representatives of the medical staff.

There is another factor that sustains the need for the medical staff search committee. Clinical leaders are inherently in an uncomfortable position at best: astraddle the fence of hospital life. One leg dangles in medical staff territory, the other in administration. It is true that a physician-leader's appointment flows ultimately from the hospital governing board through its administration, but few health care administrators are sufficiently schooled or prepared to define the credentials, background, and skills required for the job itself. Other clinicians must help to establish the thresholds of education, experience, capability, and personality needed to fill the position. For example, search committees will typically ask candidates very specific clinical questions designed to measure them against other candidates and against the specifications for the position. A prospective chief of anesthesia might be asked how he or she would handle the cancellation of a surgical case when a patient presents in the OR absent the proper laboratory values needed to proceed with the surgery. Obviously, replies to a question like this can be very technical. Such questions also frequently call for gray, rather than black-and-white, answers, and only a knowledgeable clinician can thoroughly evaluate each candidate's response.

If the search committee merits continuation, its customary strategies and tactics emphatically do not. It is a mystery why, in this fiercely competitive age, so many health care organizations haphazardly assign a disparate group of people to fill positions of vital importance to the organization and then leave them without information, direction, or limitation. This approach hardly meshes with the increasing business demands on hospitals.

The numerous, complex intertwinings of physician leadership positions and people with hospital policy, planning, politics, competitive stance, etc. may require even more savvy and stamina than high-level hospital executives and physicians can bring to the recruitment process. Attracting a "top doc" to serve as anesthesia department chair, for instance, calls for close and realistic analysis of such factors as the "market" for candidates (background, experience, compensation levels, components of an appropriate contractual agreement) in that position; the revenue stream of the hospital's existing anesthesia department; the number of CRNAs and their reporting relationship to the clinical leader (if any); and current regional practices in regard to anesthesia department management. These are issues that could be deal-breakers if not handled knowledgeably and delicately with prospective candidates for the position. This is why many medical search committees choose not to go it alone and instead seek outside assistance from search consultants.

In the past, very few hospitals have taken these kinds of issues into consideration in any depth. In fact, very few hospitals have, until recently at least, assigned a high priority to physician recruitment at all. Those that did were sporadic in their attentions—reactive more than proactive. That is, someone in the hospital typically suggested that a new product line (say, a pain clinic) be created by the institution, regardless of whether it fit the strategic plan (if there was one) or whether there was any supportable financial basis for it. The impetus was the opening of a pain clinic by a nearby hospital; the desire of the hospital's staff to have a pain clinic; or, as is all too common in health care, the fact that pain clinics are "in." So the hospital launched a search for an anesthesiologist with an interest or skill in pain management to head a pain clinic.

Such an approach does not fully focus on the development of services and the concomitant appointment of clinical leaders as a strategy for survival and prosperity. Fortunately, it is today giving way to a finer appreciation of the need to integrate these activities with the hospital's longer-range strategic plans. What we are seeing more frequently is recruitment of physicians to lead clinical product lines that stem from, and are supported by, the hospital's strategic planning process. Hence, the product lines receive the kind of financial, operational, and clinical support that they need to succeed.*

Another sign of more businesslike hospital activities is that in-house recruiters, long-entrenched in most corporations, have recently taken a seat in the administrative offices of many hospitals and health systems. Their activities are quite separate from those required of physician-leader search committees, however. Most internal physician recruiters are responsible for locating and hiring salaried, hospital-based doctors, such as house officers and primary care physicians for community-based practices. This is an important and time-consuming function, but it is an administrative one, bearing little connection to the "big picture" of the organization over time. Nor does it provide much of a basis for relationships with existing or potential "top docs." In-house recruiters seldom have the time, the understanding, or the clout to direct or redirect the activities of a "top doc" search committee effectively. Thus, search committees to locate, select, and hire candidates for clinical leadership positions will almost certainly continue, even as other aspects of health care management undergo major transformation. Whether these "tribal" groups help or hinder their organizations' growth and change is another question.

* Longshore, G. "Service Line Management/Bottom Line Management." *Journal of Health Care Finance* 24(4):72-9, Summer 1998.

CHAPTER 7

Function and Follies

The explicit functions that a modern search committee must perform are:

- <u>S</u>eek,
- <u>E</u>valuate,
- <u>A</u>nalyze,
- <u>R</u>eview, and
- <u>C</u>ommend for
- <u>H</u>ire...

a final, successful candidate for the available leadership position.

Ancient man may have counted solely on brute force to add to the clan's gene pool; modern tribal growth is done the Woody Allen way. The medical search committee process is largely cerebral, involving a good deal of thinking, planning, and individual angst. But it is also fraught with shifting group dynamics. People who are feeling their way through any critical endeavor display complexities and sensitivities. The going can be uneasy (or worse). Hidden agendas and personality quirks may pop up at any time to frustrate—even stymie—the committee's work.

In itself a booby-trapped maze of decision making, the search process is thus invariably complicated by human and organizational factors. Not all of them can be anticipated, of course, but with some preparation, most can come as less of a surprise than they usually do.

Chapter 8

Roles and Realities

The Search Committee Chair

The most critical decision for the person or entity that initiates the search for a new physician-leader is the choice of the search committee's chair. It is inestimably better not to have formed the search committee at all (and probably not to have ever filled the clinical leadership position) than to allow the process and its outcome to be directed by a chair who is not in sync with the organization's strategic plans, philosophy, and objectives. A rogue chair in a physician-leader search committee process can do more damage to a health care organization than most of its competitors.

As an appointee in a position of authority and power, the person who holds the chair will understand and represent the larger goals of the organization. A physician who chairs a search committee must, for example, find and express a balance between administrative and medical perspectives.

The chair sets the boundaries, tasks, and general tone of the search process. In essence, the chair lays the groundwork for the search committee to develop and project the organization's image throughout the life of the search. The chair may become involved in advising the hospital CEO on contractual items that he or she sees as appropriate for the potential candidate, but it is not the chair's role to develop details of any contract. Perhaps the most important function of the chair is to continuously define and reiterate the goals of the committee.

The search committee chair fills a critical communications role. He or she instructs the committee members in their responsibilities so that they clearly understand what the group should and should not do. The chair must persuade committee members that how they structure the committee can facilitate, or hamper, its work and that the mechanics of meetings and record keeping are important. Without losing sight of key details, the chair's focus on the wide, long-term organizational picture (of which the search is a part) cannot waiver.

The complexity of the search, the size of the search committee, and the chair's overall availability may dictate the need for a cochair. The cochair must act in the absence of, or in tandem with, the chair. The relationship of the role of the cochair to that of the chair needs to be clearly defined. Usually, the cochair is assigned specific, peripheral activities in support of the search committee's overall work. These might include spearheading an academic departmental review process (see Part III, Chapter 11), gathering information that will clarify the clinical responsibilities and scope of programs that exist within the department that is seeking a new physician-leader, and referencing candidates when the final field is about to be drawn.

The cochair can be the search committee representative who meets and greets candidates on their initial visits. He or she might also play host to each candidate, spouse, and family, acquainting them with the hospital and with the geographical area in which it is located.

The cochair may also be the committee member who debriefs candidates following their interviews and reports the findings back to the entire committee. In this important "linkage" position, the cochair can lobby with the committee for individual candidates' concerns. Indeed, he or she may actually negotiate nonfinancial parts of the contractual agreement when a final candidate is chosen.

Search Committee Members

Medical staff search committee members are cast in both explicit and implicit roles as the hunt for a "top doc" unfolds. The explicit role is to find and engage the best possible candidate for the job. Members depend on the chair to identify tasks and to provide them with resources to perform those tasks in pursuit of this aim. The chair depends on members to apply their knowledge, experience, and skills to the specified tasks.

The implicit function of the search committee as a whole is to provide the candidate who is eventually hired with his or her first base of support within the organization. The members may be enlisted as "salespeople" for the preferred candidate, especially if the recommendation for hiring must be reported to a separate committee of the board. Once hired, the new "top doc" is apt to need search committee members to champion his or her establishment of influence, "territory," or programs.

In this way, the search committee's implicit role complements its explicit one. The combination amounts to a strong contribution by the search committee to the type and extent of change that will shape the hospital's future. Clearly, then, the composition of the search committee (discussed in Chapter 9) is something to be considered carefully. If it isn't, half the committee's mission (the explicit half) may eventually be accomplished, but the implicit function may fail because support for the candidate weakens after hiring. To conclude a successful search, the committee must agree publicly that the new physician is, without reservation, the leader who can most effectively help the organization improve its strength, stature, and quality of performance.

There are several things that search committee members should not do. They should have no input into decisions about the form and duration of the contractual relationship between the prospective physician-leader and the organization. Nor is it within the scope of the committee's work to renegotiate or modify any contractual terms. Such concerns should remain in the CEO's bailiwick.

Management's Role

It is the health care organization's CEO who initiates the formation of a medical leadership search committee. While advice should be sought from prominent leaders of the medical staff, responsibility for appointment of the chair, and thereby control of the search committee process, should rest with the CEO.

The CEO has a responsibility to define the financial and the operational contexts within which the clinical programs under the direction of the sought-after physician-leader will take place. That is, the CEO must define the business needs that justify the appointment of this physician-leader, as well as the various programs that will be implemented under his or her direction. Some basic questions the CEO should address at the outset include:

- Is the position well-defined—are responsibilities and accountabilities clear?
- Is there enough market demand to support the clinical programs of this leader?
- Is equipment available and/or will new equipment and technology be made available to carry the programs into the future?
- Is marketing support on hand for these programs?
- Have objectives against which to measure the performance of the physician-leader once he or she is in place been set?

These and other factors that will influence the "business" of the new physician-leader need to be well-thought-out and documented by the hospital CEO before the decision to recruit is taken. They are not items that a medical search committee should be addressing, analyzing, or refining while prospective candidates come before it. But they are essential to supporting and informing the physician-leader search committee from the moment it begins its work. Without them, chances are good that the outcome will not be what is expected.

There are other important roles for the health care organization's administrative arm to play. One is to develop a framework within which the search committee can work to devise position requirements. This is a job that the board delegates to the CEO. It usually consists of a list of nonnegotiable attributes, skills, and experiences that management wants the successful candidate to possess. By establishing these parameters early and communicating them directly to the chair, the organization's leadership can bring its own agenda to the table and keep it there. This is especially useful if the CEO defers the choice of committee members to the medical staff, as may occur.

However, it can be a very delicate matter for the CEO to transmit this information to the search committee's chair without blunting the latter's enthusiasm. The CEO must get across the message that the proffered list of requirements, while permitting a fair amount of latitude in the selection process, allows no room for compromise in the selection itself. This is because the ultimate authority for appointment of a physician-leader rests not with the search committee or its chair, not with the CEO, but with the board. Unless the chosen candidate's qualifications track well with the CEO's board-directed profile, the board will not approve the selection and the search committee's months of work will have been in vain.

In two key areas, the role of the search committee should be carefully differentiated from that of the organization's leadership. These areas have to do with the actual offer of employment that will eventually be made to the agreed-upon candidate and with negotiation of a compensation and relocation package (which may include other contingencies of acceptance) with that candidate. These are emphatically not the functions of an effective search committee. Involving committee members in these aspects of the search can unleash dark forces that will, at the very least, bog down the proceedings, as will be illustrated later.

Rather, it is the responsibility of the board through the CEO, to think out, settle upon, and clearly communicate acceptable contractual agreements before the search committee process begins. These arrangements should relate to the institution's overarching framework for the appointment of physician-leaders. The CEO should stipulate an acceptable or desirable range of compensation and extras—preferably one dictated by competitive market forces. The committee's work can be done within these guidelines, with the ultimate offer of employment and associated conditions handled by the CEO and/or the CEO's designate on the committee (see Part V, Chapter 21, compensation package negotiation). While the committee's proper role is to identify and screen high-quality candidates for the available physician-leader position, it is the CEO's job to deal with the quantity aspects of negotiating the terms of employment.

Search Consultant

Before search committee members are selected and the committee itself is structured, the chair may want to consider bringing in professionals skilled and experienced in the recruitment of physician-leaders. Indeed, the CEO or another initiator of the search may engage such a professional even sooner. The reason relates to the human factors mentioned earlier. If the initiator and/or the chair can learn about some of the psychological or the professional issues that may come into play in the course of a top doc search, he or she can better manage them by choosing committee members whose needs and personalities are not apt to conflict.

Certainly the chair of a search committee in a 400-bed teaching hospital in Massachusetts would not have involved one radiation oncologist in recruiting a chief of oncology had he known what havoc that member would wreak. At least four prime candidates for the position mysteriously bowed out before the search consultant noticed a common thread running through the concerns they had expressed during regular debriefings. Upon reexamination, none was eager to point directly to the radiation oncologist as the culprit (seeing themselves as "brothers in oncology," perhaps, or worried about unpleasant repercussions). But the consultant persevered until he uncovered why this particular search committee process had "burned up" four fine candidates.
It turned out that, in private meetings, the radiation oncologist had unjustifiably criticized the clinical credentials of each of the four prospects, demeaned their chances of acceptance into the organizational culture, or otherwise discouraged them from taking the position. The chair of this particular search committee was in firm control, however, and once the problem was identified, he was able to alter the interview process so that no more member-candidate meetings took place out-

side his presence. However, 12 months and four candidates had been lost to the radiation oncologist's apparent fear of losing the hospital's oncology "spotlight" to the person chosen for the chief of oncology position. It took six more months to complete the search.

An experienced search consultant with special knowledge of physician-leader recruitment brings invaluable insights to the search committee, including information about local, regional, and specialty-specific trends toward salaried, fee-for-service, or hybrid compensation arrangements between health care organizations and various types of physician-leaders. A search committee needs to know such things before it strikes out in one direction or another. For instance, until a few years ago, unless the hospital was serving a heavy Medicare and/or indigent population, a chief of emergency medicine in most metropolitan areas would not accept a salaried employment arrangement; fee-for-service billing, an administrative stipend, and independence were required items for most candidates for a chief of emergency medicine position. Now, because of the influence of managed care and capitated arrangements, most chiefs of emergency medicine are very happy with salaried arrangements. Pathologists are also moving toward salaried arrangements as inpatient revenue and related diagnostic testing are further restricted by the influence of managed care contracting. Working alone, a search committee cannot hope to duplicate this sort of broad and up-to-date knowledge of marketplace conditions.

A physician-leader search consultant will be able to advise a search committee on the supply-and-demand issues related to physician specialty, as well as on programs and amenities that need to be in place in order to attract the best candidates. The latter might include marketing and other practice support and data from administration and from existing specialty and subspecialty staff, and information about equipment available, caseloads, and referral patterns that will compliment or enhance the new physician-leader's practice. These are factors that tend to be ignored by search committees working on their own until late in the process, when they are either considered in a rush or, more likely, cause the process to bog down. By preparing the committee for such issues well before they arise, the search consultant can also make the organization look good to the market—like an institution with clear and soundly supported direction in its clinical programs.

Although "early" is the best time to seek assistance from a properly qualified search consultant (for more on qualifications, see Part I, Chapter 5), our experience has been that most medical staff search committee members have already been appointed by the time we are invited onto the scene. Nonetheless, the search firm can do a great deal to help from this point on.

- It can help to formulate a detailed position specification (or refine one already developed by the search's initiator and/or the committee chair), submitting it for critical review and final approval to the search committee.
- It can serve as a lightning rod, deflecting the heat of discussions about the appropriate qualifications, skills, and experiences for the right candidate. The consultant can take the heat off the CEO and the search committee chair when tough decisions have to be made.
- It can, and should, act as liaison in the development of well-qualified candidates, in contacting them, and in managing their interactions with the committee.

- As the recruitment process unfolds, it can serve as a highly effective debriefer of candidates, whose feedback is likely to flow more easily to a consultant than to a search committee member. In addition, what candidates have to say during these debriefings often suggests valuable mid-course corrections in the position specification. The consultant is able to discern, analyze, and make constructive use of this information.

- It can advise and assist in closing the best deal with the candidate.

Another role for the search consultant—one that hospitals may not initially contemplate—is marketer for the institution and its programs. In the course of marketing the open position, the consultant will be in contact with residency program directors, heads of professional societies, trade organizations, deans, and chairs of major departments in academic medical centers. While search committee members and the organization, through its advertising, are expected to describe the institution in glowing terms, an outside party often has a credibility edge. This is particularly true if the third party's knowledge and accomplishments are respected throughout the health care industry.

A search consultant's involvement generally means that the most critical function of the search committee is reserved for its members, while the search firm fills a number of auxiliary roles without which the assignment cannot be completed. That is, the consultant improves the efficiency of the search committee process and the number and quality of the candidates presented for consideration. The main job of the committee is to review, interview, and evaluate those speedily produced, first-rate candidates.

The consultant will save the health care organization both time and money in its search for a new physician-leader. Over the 18 months of the aforementioned chief of oncology search, for instance, the community hospital involved lost significant ground to competitors. While its search moved ahead at glacial speed, nearby hospitals were developing their own oncology programs—with leaders for them already in place. And those physician-leaders were busy attracting patients and cementing their institutions' relationships with community hospitals to help them market specialized oncology services and with academic medical centers at the forefront of oncology research.

Time and time again, in corporate and not-for-profit settings alike, it has been an "outside expert" who has enlivened a moribund task force. Reputable consultants come with instant credibility—a solid track record of achieving for others just what a medical staff search committee wants to achieve for itself.

Chapter 9

Selection and Structure

Choosing the Chair

Selecting the person who will shepherd the committee through the search process is second only in importance to choosing the best candidate for the available position. This is no exaggeration. Whether it is the CEO who names the chair (as is preferable), the board chair, or the president of the medical staff, the time taken to contemplate a number of factors will prove to be well-spent.

A good place to begin is with a review of the roles the chair may play (see Part II, Chapter 8). Reflect upon how the backgrounds, temperaments, and workloads of the individuals under consideration might mesh with such responsibilities. Also important are possible political ramifications of certain appointments. The chair must be able to rise above interests of any stripe—economic, territorial, generational, etc.—that may conflict with the main objectives of the search.

Look for an individual who has a facilitative, rather than a dominative, style of leadership, as well as a flair for administration. The chair must be the sort of person who can capitalize on the group's tendencies toward consonance and conformity. When sticking points cause delay, it is the chair who will have to act as arbitrator, confronting committee members' biases, steering debate away from narrow concerns, and focusing attention on the organization's larger, long-term interests.

Because the chair is the navigator of an often-tricky course, it is advantageous if he or she has had prior search committee experience. Someone with a successful track record in this area has already demonstrated both the capability and the perseverance required to complete a search committee's jobs.

The wrong choice of chair has doomed more than a few health care executive searches. Disinterested or overextended chairs, for example, have led search committees into, but not out of, the woods. This is what happened when the board of a major East Coast academic medical center sought a new vice president for engineering to deal with a plague of power outages that had repeatedly crippled hospital functions. The board formed a multidisciplinary search committee, but, from the beginning, the search was loosely organized and loosely chaired. At first, the committee members attended luncheon meetings and enthusiastically joined in discussions of the experience and background needed for the position. Varied and shifting views were exchanged, but the meetings went on without a push for consensus from the chair.

Eventually, the debate wore thin, and, after 10 months and 10 candidates, even lunch was not a sufficient enticement to committee members. As they realized that they were aiming at a moving target, they began to remove themselves from the committee one by one. In the eleventh month, the remaining members, exhausted and demoralized, recommended for hire a candidate whom they had not evaluated thoroughly. He became the new engineering vice president, but, nine months later, the hospital was still experiencing power blackouts. In the tenth month after his last-gasp hiring, the new vice president was terminated.

In appointing a search committee chair, consider whether the prospective leader:

- Understands and agrees with the business goals and the strategic direction of the organization.
- Has a sincere interest in having the search committee produce the best possible candidate for the organization.
- Is prepared to voice his or her honest opinion to the committee on all occasions, no matter what the cost.
- Is organized and able to organize others.
- Can assimilate large amounts of information and synthesize it for clear, concise feedback.
- Is aware of the approximately four to 12 months required to complete a physician-leadership search and can dedicate that amount of time to it.
- Is prepared to facilitate group consensus, including deferring personal biases for or against a candidate to the majority opinion of the committee.
- Is an adroit manager of conflict.
- Has a secretary, or access to one, who can support the search process.
- Has no conflict of interest or competitive concerns that could color opinions of certain candidates.
- Has chaired or participated in a successful prior search.

Appointing the Members

Ideally, the chair will have a free hand in planning the composition of the search committee to achieve a balanced knowledge and power base (see Appendix 2 for sample search committee structures). In some cases, the hospital's administration and/or the board of trustees may intervene in membership selection. More often, the medical staff will have substantial input at this stage, either by virtue of the hospital's by-laws, which may require medical staff approval of committee members; the CEO's or the chair's gesture of courtesy in requesting medical staff review and approval of members; or simple preemption by medical staff people. As mentioned earlier, no recruitment of a physician-leader can be expected to go forward fruitfully without firm support from the organization's medical staff.

The chief search committee "talent scout"—generally the chair—should seek diverse members from a cross-section of the organization. People who are viewed as knowledgeable and influential leaders in their areas are the most desirable. Unfortunately, this is not the way that search committee membership selection usually proceeds.

It is currently common practice to choose a homogeneous medical staff search committee from among a closed group or clique: the "old boys." Yet this approach has repeatedly proved detrimental to the job at hand. It tends to encourage factional infighting that diverts attention away from organizational objectives and toward challenging the chair's authority. Such bickering can destroy a search committee. At best, it causes the less fractious members to behave passively, desiring nothing more than to escape the committee. Should a prolonged, fruitless search lead to the appearance of a search consultant, the "old boys" will usually disapprove. They persist in believing that their way is the best way, even though the results they've produced fly in the face of this contention.

If a search committee becomes more concerned with its internal dynamics than with its assignment, it should be disbanded. Like the one assembled to locate a new chair of surgery for a 500-bed inner-city teaching hospital, it won't accomplish anything anyway. This committee spent more time arguing over the clinical training that candidates shouldn't have than they did seeking candidates. Some members of the committee were intent on keeping vascular surgeons, who would directly compete with them, out of the candidate pool. After two years and no candidates, the committee was dissolved. A strong chair would have cut off such diversionary—and divisive—tactics by pointing back to the pre-approved position specification's non-exclusion of vascular surgeons as candidates.

Earlier, the role of search committee members in helping the newly hired physician-leader to assimilate into the hospital organization was discussed. This should be a key consideration as committee members are chosen, for the "power base" represented by those members should facilitate, not impede, assimilation. However, the chair should take care to choose committee members who, above all, have the best interests of the hospital at heart and who can cut through their own agendas or needs in fulfillment of those interests.

Search committee members should be willing and able to contribute their time actively to a process that can extend over many months. Most serve voluntarily, but an astute chair or CEO can "prime" certain desirable physicians so that they are eager to participate in just the right search. The process of selecting search committee members is usually quite informal, taking place in hallways and cafeterias, so those in a position to know that a search is imminent can probe and prod potential committee members about their willingness to serve.

There are physicians who volunteer a tad *too* vigorously for search committee work. When someone seems overly anxious to participate, the chair and/or CEO should be cautious, for it is likely that that person has a hidden agenda and seeks to control the search committee process to satisfy it.

Approached at the right time and in the right way, the most potentially productive members for any given search committee will often agree to work together. This obviously improves the organization's chances of completing a successful search in short order. Traditionally, each designated committee member is notified informally of his or her appointment by the chair and then is formally contacted about the time and place of the first committee meeting.

Structuring the Search Committee

The deliberate, well-organized approach that characterizes most hospitals' searches for CEOs is not matched in their attempts to locate clinical leaders. This relates to the traditional "old boy network" method, which lends itself to a haphazard search committee structure even when a top doc position needs to be filled.

Those experienced in recruiting clinical leaders know that the membership and the size of the committee play a major part in how it will function. Large committees tend toward complicated group dynamics that can confuse and frustrate the purposes of the search. This could be seen in the previously described vice president for engineering search, which was mounted by a committee of 21.

Coordinating individuals' schedules and building and solidifying consensus are more easily accomplished with a few than with a multitude. The greater the number of members, the higher the probability that the process will carry on beyond the projected time frame; restricting committee size increases committee effectiveness. The most effective search committees has six to eight members.

When this committee size is not feasible or politic, and a dozen or more people become involved in the search committee's work, a smaller subcommittee is recommended. This "steering committee," consisting of no more than four people (possibly including the chair and/or cochair and other prominent members of the committee), should have the task of carrying out the parent group's directives. It might take on the majority of the responsibility for the search, reporting out only those candidates who survive its own screening process.

Finally, once a search committee is formed, it is best to preserve its original composition. Adding new members after meetings have begun and procedures are under way will only upset the group's dynamics.

Some examples of how physician-leader search committees might be structured in various types of hospitals are shown in Appendix 2

TOP DOCS

Part III

The Search Committee Process

CHAPTER 10

The Influence of the Organization

In the quest for a key physician, the roles of the medical staff search committee—both the overt and the implicit ones—remain the same regardless of the sort of health care organization involved. However, the committee process is affected by the type of hospital seeking a top doc.

Academic medical centers (where bylaws commonly stipulate that a search committee must be formed when certain faculty-level positions are open) and tertiary care institutions tend to rely heavily on the traditional "old boy" network in their medical staff searches. Search committee members in a teaching hospital are likely to be faculty appointees who chair the most important departments—"old boys" who are supremely confident that they know the precise clinical, academic, and personal background and experience that the "new boy" must have to fit in. Therefore, these search committee members are primarily looking for a candidate who is as much like them as possible. They have probably not worked with a search firm in the past and are not apt to welcome one into the process now. It is important to such a committee to exert strong and sustained control over the entire search process.

The teaching or research-oriented hospital must devise a double set of standards—clinical and academic—for its prospective physician-leaders. It usually has in hand a faculty practice plan to help. With so many criteria already existing, the search committee seldom perceives a need for more information derived from market data, such as the appropriate level of compensation for a physician comparable to the one it seeks. Overall, the "business" implications and benefits of hiring one candidate instead of another tend to escape academic and tertiary care institutions. As more and more such hospitals experience fiscal problems, of course, these blinders will fall off.

A community hospital's medical staff search committee may behave similarly in some cases. However, its membership is probably more representative of its organization as a whole than the membership of a typical academic or tertiary care institution's medical staff search committee. A cross-section of medical and administrative staff and trustees is likely to make up the search committee of a community hospital. Absent the academic institution's traditional requirements and faculty practice plan as a framework, such a committee is likely to look willingly to a search consultant for help in developing specifications for the available position. It may well depend almost exclusively on the search firm's advice about the appropriate education, experience, personal attributes, and compensation for the physician it wants to hire. It will certainly ask the firm to produce all or almost all of the candidates.

It's not that the "old boy" network isn't alive and well in the community hospital setting, but its importance has been eroded by marketplace pressures on community hospitals. Still, it can stir conflict in the search committee process in any hospital where it takes precedence.

In contrast to most not-for-profit institutions, proprietary institutions (and for-profit organizations in general) have a much better idea of what they want *before* they mount a search. They have identified their business needs far in advance, and they tend to develop very concrete educational and professional specifications, as well as definite ideas about the "chemistry" needed to meet those requirements. Many not-for-profit hospitals, for example, will not have considered current or projected income streams for the department for which they seek a new physician-leader. A search firm will frequently create such income statements for not-for-profit hospitals (see Appendix 3), only to have them greeted with a yawn by administrators who simply do not know how important these data are to their search and to their institution's ability to compete.

It is important to understand that, regardless of the type of hospital involved, health care institutions lag well behind corporate America when it comes to leadership search. They have caught up significantly in the area of administrative executive recruitment, but the entire process of finding and appointing physician-leaders still comprises a big black hole of misunderstanding and mismanagement in most hospitals.

The physician side of the business is not well understood by many hospital CEOs, and hospitals are not paying as much attention to developing and running efficient search committees as they should. The outcome is that most physician-leader searches continue to be controlled by physicians, who use the "old boy" network in a frequently disorganized and untargeted effort to locate candidates. This situation does not serve contemporary hospitals well. If they are to survive and be profitable in the future, it has to change.

CHAPTER 11

Departmental Review Process

Historically, the departmental review has been an extensive, periodic analysis and decision-making process that originated in academic medical centers but can be used by—and be similarly valuable to—any sizable hospital, particularly community teaching hospitals and health systems with academic relationships. It is a process that examines the clinical, research, educational, financial, and administrative aspects of a department, thereby highlighting the interrelationships among them.

Involving both internal and outside reviewers, the process has traditionally been designed to gauge whether a department's policies and programs are cogent, effective, and in tune with the hospital's mission. Departmental reviews of the 1970s and 1980s resulted in better evaluations of departmental productivity, more strategic approaches to long-range planning, and more businesslike management of resources than in the past.

However, the benefits of these reviews have been offset by a variety of problems that chafe leaders of health care institutions. "The way departmental reviews are usually done is a very inefficient process that often does not yield the desired outcomes," in the view of a former academic medical center executive in Philadelphia. Another senior executive, this one based at a mid-Atlantic university hospital, notes that "the politicization of departmental reviews compromises their effectiveness." And a health care consultant who was formerly an academic medical center executive said, "The traditional departmental review is no longer relevant to contemporary issues and pressures within the health care industry."

Politics is an example of one vexing problem. Because many of the data and much of the analysis of a traditional departmental review are generated internally, a political subtext weaves its way through the process. Even the value of outside reviewers is somewhat mitigated by logistical problems. And too much time between traditional reviews leaves institutions out of step with the rapid changes taking place in the nation's health care system.

The advent of the 21st Century calls for a more timely and precise understanding of the content and quality of each academic hospital department. The proportionate roles and priorities of clinical care, research, and education, and a workable view of how each sector will provide its own resources, need to be spelled out. For both fiduciary and programmatic purposes, an objective and realistic "valuation" needs to be placed on all departments involved in the integrated health care systems of the future.

The Eight Components of a Departmental Review

Today, health care institutions need to come to grips with how they will handle departmental reviews in a highly volatile environment. A contemporary departmental review should:

- Measure the human and the physical resources of a department.
- Provide a clear picture of the organization of each hospital department, showing how effectively all its components function.
- Point up the strengths and the weaknesses of each organizational area.
- Suggest the best strategic utilization of resources for the future.
- Demonstrate how each area of the organization is accommodating changes in today's health care system.
- Develop an insightful profile of a department that can facilitate current or future searches for new leadership.
- Create, prospectively, a readily available resource for strategizing the consolidation of departments as integrated networks are developed.
- Establish a system for acquiring and maintaining information that can be used as a resource for decision making well beyond the review itself.

While a traditional departmental review generally meets the first four requirements, it seldom satisfies the last four to any great extent. The last four should be included because they are increasingly important in keeping hospitals from being swept away by the tides of change.

Advantages of the Contemporary Departmental Review

The contemporary approach varies from the traditional departmental review in several important ways.

1. **It takes into consideration funding, marketplace, and regulatory issues that significantly affect the institution and suggests how a department can effectively address them.** In addition to evaluating the content and quality of clinical, educational, and research programs in each department, it defines the direction that each departmental component should take in accordance with current funding trends. These issues are increasingly crucial to hospitals' survival; for instance, Moody's bond rating service recently downgraded the bonds of some hospitals and health care systems that were deemed to lack effective departmental mergers.

2. **It streamlines the complicated process of selecting the most capable leaders.** Recruiting objective, discreet, willing, and energetic review committee members and chairs who can devote a considerable amount of time to the project has historically been an internal process. A member of the institution's senior management team chooses a chair of the review committee from senior physicians and/or faculty. The committee chair and the dean or chief executive officer meet with the chair of the department to be reviewed, seeking consensus on the goals, cooperative efforts, and scheduling of the review process.

   In the contemporary approach to departmental review, the organization of the review committee, its activities, and its scheduling are often facilitated by a knowledgeable outside consulting resource. This not only speeds up the process, but also helps ensure that, from the outset, the chair has the assistance of a consultant with a demonstrable grasp of trends in the field and an understanding of how a department's efforts need to be synchronized with those trends.

   Especially in academic medical centers, the person who chairs the review committee becomes the chair of the search committee for a new departmental leader. To say it another way, the departmental review committee becomes the search committee when a new departmental leader is required. Therefore, if the appointment of a new departmental chair or leader is anticipated, it would be wise to have the chair of the review committee review the recommendation in Part II, Chapters 8 and 9, of this book when selecting committee members.

3. **It overcomes the inefficiencies inherent in an internally conducted review.** Traditional reviews distract valuable professional and staff personnel and take up enormous amounts of time that could be used more productively. This is especially true for the tedious job of data-gathering and reporting. Many people at the divisional and departmental levels must spend time amassing large amounts of data from diverse sources that a review requires. It is often much more cost-effective for an outside consultant, focusing on nothing but the review itself, to collect targeted data and then to develop and present the background material. Experienced consultants will take only 20 percent of the time it would take the department's personnel to collect data and report them in an analyzable format.

4. **It avoids political pitfalls.** Peer review of departments will inevitably involve judgments that are subjective at best and politically motivated at worst. This bias can be substantially reduced through independent production and analysis of data and information pertinent to a contemporary review.

   The objectivity of outside consultants typically lends credibility to the process, and it will help the committee chair to develop a clear set of objectives for existing and new programs that extend over several years, and then to integrate those goals into a strategic plan for the department as a whole.

5. **It can improve the external review part of the process.** Once the internal review report is completed, it becomes the key source document for external peer reviewers who have been retained to assess the department. The report can be sent to reviewers in advance of their site visit, and it can serve as a backdrop for the outside reviewers' meetings, discussions, and final written report to the hospital committee chair. This approach speeds up the external reviewers' process and allows them to focus more precisely on the issues they need to examine during their on-site visit.

6. **It provides a post-review legacy of accessible information.** This legacy has several potential uses and benefits. It can be used to establish benchmarks by which the performance of department chairs can be evaluated. It can provide easily maintained information to be used in strategic and operational planning. And it can serve as the baseline for full departmental reviews in the future, or for interim audits between full reviews. These would include objectives in clinical, administrative, and relationship-building areas that, ideally, would devolve from outcomes measures.

7. **It provides a map for a newly recruited physician leader to lead the department to achieve its goals.** The departmental review report is an especially useful tool for the new chair to use in redirecting the department and enables the leader to hit the ground running. It also allows the health care organization's CEO or dean to track and measure the new chair's progress and accomplishments. This will be helpful in the payment of incentive compensation and bonus awards.

Triggers and Timing

The decision to conduct a departmental review is usually made by the dean of an academic institution or by the CEO of a medical center. Not all departments are reviewed at once; a staggered schedule of reviews generally stretches over two to three years.

When a new CEO or dean joins a health care organization, or when there is a change in the leadership of a department or division, people's expectations of and requirements for a departmental review are likely to change. New leaders may undertake more or less rigorous reviews than their predecessors. But many will welcome reviews early in their tenure in order to identify problems, to formulate possible solutions, and to track results.

Whenever they are done, departmental reviews should serve to rouse hospital staff out of their usual routines by requiring them to take a fresh look at themselves. Most academic and community teaching hospital departments have historically been reviewed every four to six years—too infrequently, we believe, for the fast-moving pace of contemporary medicine. Although many institutions might find a greater frequency onerous, there is no underestimating the ongoing impact of changes in the health care industry when considering departmental performance and value.

By and large, most sizable hospitals and health care systems will benefit by beginning with an all-encompassing review of each department and then conducting less intensive reviews every one to two years. Databases should be briefly audited and updated annually and thoroughly reviewed every two years. Every three or four years, another full departmental review is recommended.

Special events may also trigger a full departmental review. They include:

- A shift in organizational, departmental, or divisional leadership.
- An anticipated merger, alliance, or network integration.
- A search for new departmental leadership.
- A follow-up to a major institutional or systemwide reorganization.
- A major program expansion requiring special input.

Impact of Health Industry Changes: Funding

Continuing changes in funding, marketplace, and regulatory areas are having the most significant effects on the departmental review process. Academic medical centers, their affiliated hospitals, and community teaching hospitals are especially vulnerable to the vagaries of health care financing.

Managed care is forcing cutbacks in research and teaching, as well as delays in trials of new therapies. The financial pressures increase wherever the buying power of managed care organizations is ascendant. For years, teaching hospitals have relied on a varied array of funding sources (including Washington, D.C., and state capitals) that is now dissipating. The federal government is reducing its commitment to graduate medical education (GME) at the same time that MCOs disclaim any responsibility for GME financing. Managed care's renowned penny-pinching has now penetrated the Medicare and Medicaid programs. Teaching hospitals have lost their ability to shift GME costs among payers as they depend more on the global payment streams that reflect MCOs' risk pools. Who will be left to pay for the expensive educations of tomorrow's physicians? The answer may lie in some combination of government funding and self-financing by students. Both sources represent funds for which hospitals will have to compete.

To vie successfully for the limited dollars that are available, a hospital must have a clearer picture of the sources and uses of its revenues than a traditional departmental review usually offers. In academic medical centers and community teaching hospitals, where complex interdependencies often develop in response to diverse financial pressures, a contemporary review can tease apart these relationships and then be used to hone a department's competitive edge.

Another funding issue is related to technology and its transfer out of academic medicine and into applied research. The money required to meet the demand for new technology outstrips the ability of most hospitals to raise funds quickly. To accommodate this situation, teaching hospitals need to focus their research in new ways. For example, innovations related to patient outcomes measurements may attract the funding support of MCOs.

Indeed, if a hospital's or department's research isn't moving to the physician's office or the bedside these days, the chances of eliciting financial support are diminished.

Contemporary departmental reviews can address the extent to which medicine should be influenced by commercial interests—an important question with which health care providers are wrestling. By highlighting an institution's resources and commitments, a contemporary departmental review can pinpoint the locations of various research projects, suggest which research is marketable, and propose ways for the institution to advance those projects and the people involved with them. Without interfering with the research itself, such a review can often help the hospital develop better strategies for using it.

Impact of Health Industry Changes: Marketplace Issues

Resources are expanding as hospitals and health care systems acquire more and more assets through mergers, acquisitions, and system development.

While optimizing these resources is the ideal, it is often difficult, if not impossible, to sort them out. A contemporary review of departments in merging hospitals can clarify how they will fit together. It can help shape or reshape departments in accordance with market forces by relating marketplace information to the hospital's internal circumstances and strategies.

On the whole, few department chiefs (especially in academic medical centers) understand how to tie resource planning for patient care to marketplace opportunities or constraints. They often have only a limited grasp of which lines of service should be emphasized, how to price services, or how to negotiate profitably with payers within the payment structure. To help department chiefs in their strategic planning, a consulting resource experienced in facilitating departmental reviews can collect and digest information about broad market forces that affect the department's operations.

Impact of Health Industry Changes: Regulatory Issues

Hospital CEOs would like their department chairs to be more accountable for administrative, supervisory, and teaching (AS&T) activities. The federal government is beginning to respond to fraud and abuse in this area with oversight audits that require hospitals to document that compensation of chairs and program directors is related to the actual time they spend on AS&T. A contemporary departmental review can quantify that time, as well as other time spent on nonclinical activities, thereby providing a structure for compliance with these regulations and oversight audits.

In fact, the contemporary departmental review should prepare hospitals for all the regulatory and accreditation reviews they must undergo. The "legacy system" left behind by professional departmental review consultants is a database that can be drawn upon, and built upon, for this purpose.

Results of a Contemporary Review

A hospital or health care system should expect specific and substantial results from a contemporary departmental review:

- A sharp picture of how the department is organized and the level of function within each division.
- A concise record of the strengths and weaknesses in each departmental area.
- An analysis of the department's accommodations to the changes occurring in the health care industry.
- A "legacy" database that, beyond the review itself, can be built upon and used for performance evaluations, regulatory compliance, and programmatic decision making.
- A set of concrete recommendations to aid in strategic planning for the future.

As the 21st Century arrives, it will be increasingly easy for the organization to update the database internally, although it will still need an objective, outside eye to assess the information in terms of external influences from funding sources, the marketplace, and regulators.

CHAPTER 12

Political Considerations

Health care institutions find themselves in the thick of politics from the very outset of a search for a new leader. As we have seen, it is not uncommon for both the hospital CEO and the medical staff to lobby for appointment of search committee members who reflect their own aims and desires, however they may diverge from overall organizational objectives.

The political issues surrounding the search for a new physician-leader may be legion, but, alas, they are not always apparent. They may not seem to affect the search until it is well under way or even nearing conclusion, as in the case of the "ornery oncologist" cited earlier. It is the unenviable job of the initiator and/or chair of the medical staff search committee to ferret out political time bombs and defuse them before they can maim or destroy the search committee's work.

The best time to do so is before committee members are appointed. Indeed, it is something to be considered even before the chair is named, for a chair with a hidden agenda or a vested interest in the outcome of a search can undermine—in the short or the long run—a search committee's work. A recent example involved a chief of orthopedic surgery (a division of the hospital's department of surgery) who was appointed to preside over a search for a new chair and residency program director for the department of surgery. The chief wanted the job himself, but, by virtue of his specialty, was not eligible to be a residency program director. To offset this obstacle, he convinced the search committee to hire a new department chair who would make *him* look good. That is, the new hire was an effective residency director, but was not capable of leading the department of surgery in other programmatic initiatives. The result was an ineffective chair who had to be replaced just two years later. In the meantime, the hospital's surgical service initiatives suffered. Needless to say, what was good for the Section Chief of Orthopedics was not good for the hospital.

A thoughtful chair will spend time anticipating who might bring what conflicting interests to the search process and whether and how any of these interests might undermine the committee's explicit and implicit functions. Had the chair of a Miami hospital's search for a top doc considered carefully the implications of appointing a certain pulmonologist to the committee, he would have escaped a political quagmire that caused a six-month delay. In this case, the best candidate for the available chair of medicine position was a trained and practicing pulmonologist. Despite the candidate's stellar credentials, the search committee's pulmonologist argued vigorously against him. His opposition stemmed from competitive jaundice regarding the practice of pulmonology. Although it was some time before he could be persuaded to approve the favored candidate, he eventually rallied to the majority opinion in the face of his colleagues' unassailable support for that individual. Additionally, he became one of the newly hired chair's best friends and staunchest supporters.

A political expression of professional jealousies may also hinder a search committee's work when the new physician-leader is to be offered an array of financial and practice-related supports by the hospital. Many search committee members are likely to have given fairly long service to the hospital, having started their own practices alone, with little or no help from the institution. Envious of the ease with which the new doctor will slip into a leadership position—and, like the Miami pulmonologist, of how readily he or she can compete directly with them for patients—these committee members may sabotage the search and/or the incoming physician's successful assimilation into the organization.

Another political issue that may relate to the history and length of service of many search committee members has to do with discussion of the prospective physician-leader's compensation. Especially if the recruited physician represents a specialty area that is in high demand and low supply, talk of compensation among the search committee members can quickly turn political. Take, for instance, the field of perinatology—one in which a physician who has just completed a fellowship can easily be paid more than $200,000 a year. (See Part V for more details on "top doc" compensation research.) An experienced chief of perinatology in a mid-sized hospital could receive a minimum of $350,000 in annual cash compensation. Some physicians on the search committee may be paid half or less of what such newcomers can command.

It's easy to see why they might turn pay into a political football as they go about recruiting, screening, and approving someone who will be their professional "peer." Keeping this football out of the game is the only way to deflate it, which is why we strongly recommend that compensation not be an issue on the medical staff search committee's agenda. Rather, it should be dealt with only by the chair and/or an administrative representative of the organization prior to and during the search.

Another political problem can arise not from the amount of compensation, but from the form that compensation takes. Controversy commonly erupts when a community hospital decides to recruit its first salaried physician-leader. The trend toward salaries for physicians in hospital leadership positions is inexorable, but many entrenched department chiefs and staff physicians still disparage it as "the corporatization of medicine." A good deal of a search committee's time may thus be spent wrangling over this issue if the hospital has not openly discussed and solicited consensus on it before the committee's work begins. Even if a committee so divided can agree on a candidate for the available position, that person will not begin his or her job with solid support from all committee members. Hence, while its explicit tasks will have been completed, the search committee will have failed to perform its implicit role. Another search effort may have to be undertaken if the new physician-leader is unable to overcome this barrier to assimilation.

An experienced physician-leader search firm should be able to help identify most of the potential political problems following its initial information-gathering efforts. These include interviews with the search committee as a whole and/or individual members, meetings with appropriate administrative staff representatives, and a review of background materials. The consultant should discuss likely obstacles with the chair, and, together, they should map out a way to present and discuss them in the early committee meetings.

Having the search consultant describe potential political problems in writing to the search committee is recommended. The written word lends these concerns the kind of weight and substance that demand a response from committee members. That response will suggest to the consultant the best problem-solving tack. Further, a written document will signal those in higher places *outside* the search committee that some extra influence might be helpful in eliminating a political issue. A cardiologist serving on a search committee seeking a new chief of medicine might, for example, want to discourage recruitment of another cardiologist for the post. A written statement to this effect would alert the chair, the president of the medical staff, and the hospital's CEO to the committee member's need for direct reassurance that the new physician-leader will not be allowed any clinical practice that would adversely affect the cardiologist's practice. Thus assuaged, the cardiologist should bring an open mind to the search.

The aim is to air all agendas and to resolve thorny issues before candidates enter the picture. Candidates who become aware that such political problems are part of the deliberation over their employment are bound to feel imperiled and may drop out of the running. Early grappling with the politics inherent in the search committee's processes and people can help to avoid potentially far-reaching problems. Granted, this preliminary task may not be appealing to hard-pressed search chairs. But a thorough exploration of the political issues that *can* be foreseen before the committee's work commences will leave them time and energy. And they will need time and energy to deal with the unforeseeable issues that may well arise in the course of the search.

CHAPTER 13

Groundwork by the Chair

Before the search committee has even met, the chair will have been involved in the various preliminaries discussed in previous chapters. The eventual success of the search committee's efforts is closely akin to the savvy, sensitivity and stick-to-it-iveness with which the chair pursues these early activities. It is also tied to the way in which the chair lays the groundwork for the search prior to, and during, the committee's initial meeting.

A physician-leader search committee assembled for the very first time is not yet a team. However carefully chosen, members are, by and large, physicians. And physicians tend, by nature, to be highly individualistic—not group animals at all. They may have tribal allegiance, but not yet to this sub-tribe. Generally, they are more accustomed to being team leaders than team players; more used to having others leap unquestioningly to their commands than to the slower give-and-take of consensus-building; more comfortable with being in control than with being told what to do. It is up to the chair to knit these disparate individuals into a sturdy fabric and to keep the group actively united in a common purpose—all the while expecting that a previously invisible seam will rip open.

Most search committee members arrive at that first meeting with a genuine desire to participate fully. An atmosphere of goodwill prevails, and there is a natural inclination toward concord. Too bad it doesn't last.

Many of these well-meaning folks will become frustrated with the nuts-and-bolts of recruiting and hiring a physician-leader, even though they recognize intellectually that a number of tedious steps are necessarily part of an effective search. They may begin to skip meetings, or pay scant attention to those they attend. This is especially true when searches drag on, as they often do. Committee members may become exasperated if promising candidates drop out of contention. Just to get it over with, the committee may end up settling for something less than the best possible candidate.

Avoiding the worst of these possible conditions depends to a large extent on the chair's ability to plan and lead a search that both committee members and candidates will perceive as well-managed. As important as the chair's big-picture perspective is, pulling off a well-managed search requires equal skill in the nuts-and-bolts. From the first moment of the first meeting, the chair's administrative talents will be tested by seemingly minor details that can play a major role in determining the outcome of the search.

Time, place, and frequency of meetings are among these details. Attendance will be spotty if meeting schedules or sites too often inconvenience members. While initial organizational meetings could last an hour or two, subsequent regular meetings should run no longer than an hour to an hour and a half. (Meetings preceded by a meal could last up to ninety minutes). Meetings that run beyond these thresholds may well bore committee members. As was noted by Douglas and Baker, "Ask people to name their greatest time wasters, and you'll find meetings near the top of their list."*

When scheduling meetings, the chair should strive to keep the time of day and the meeting place consistent. Once meetings get under way, the schedules should be followed despite the inevitable blandishments of individual members. Early breakfast or lunch meetings usually boost attendance, especially if food is served. Committee members see mealtime scheduling as a gesture that is supportive of their need to carry on with their other responsibilities.

The chair should arrange ahead of time for the minutes of each meeting to be recorded, not just for absentees to read, but also to document the search process. A word of caution regarding published minutes—be certain you do not leave a ticking bomb in the files to explode later. The published minutes of a medical school search committee evaluating candidates for Chair of Physical Medicine and Rehabilitation contained the following statement: "The members of the committee were unanimous in their support of Dr. Johnson's candidacy but also agreed that he was too old." In the event this candidate does not get the nod as the new Chair of PM&R, an age discrimination investigation could cost this medical school millions.

The published minutes will come in handy when the inevitable moments of confusion, disagreement or ignorance arise. Reviewing them can quickly set the record straight, enabling the committee to move on with

its real tasks. Additionally, any "housekeeping" matters handled by the chair should be duly noted in the minutes, so that the committee members are kept informed. At each formal committee meeting, the minutes of the prior meeting should be read and accepted, according to Robert's Rules of Order. (See Appendix 4.)

The chair needs to harness the group's attention and respect at the first meeting by addressing the five "W's":

- Why are we here?
- What are we here to do?
- When are we going to do it?
- Where are we going to do it?
- Who are we going to seek?

Douglas, M., and Baker, L. *The New Time Management*. Niles, Ill.: Nightingale-Conant, 1986.

To assist in laying this groundwork before the committee at its first meeting, we advise the chair to prepare as follows:

- Draft a position specification for the search in relation to the goals of the organization. Particular attention should be paid to the "responsibilities" and "requirements" sections. (See the example in Appendix 5.) You may need to reiterate this statement throughout the search to keep the committee on track.
- Plan a welcome for all members of the team, along with a summary introduction of each member's background (if they don't already know each other very well).
- Develop a general overview of the search effort—its steps and time frame—to deliver at the initial meeting. Include references to the strategic work plan and to deadlines. (See Part III, Chapter 14, for details on this.)
- Arrange for the meeting site and schedule meetings beforehand, then announce where and when the group will meet on a regular basis. Some chairs may want to seek consensus on times and place, but most will benefit from calculating what's convenient to the majority before the first meeting and then simply announcing the schedule.
- Plan to have minutes of every meeting summarized and promptly distributed to members.
- Establish and communicate the ground rules for conduct of meetings based on Robert's Rules of Order.
- Think out approaches to the target market of candidates and present them to the committee.

In addition, the chair should be prepared to deal with the following agenda items at the committee's initial meeting.

- Set forth the decision-making processes that will be followed (e.g., majority or unanimous vote; secret or open ballot in writing or by show of hands).
- If the committee's size warrants a cochair and/or steering committees (each of which should have its own leader, sub-goals, and timetable), be prepared to assign them at the first meeting.
- Tell members what they won't be permitted to do. For example, members should understand that they may not reveal the identity of candidates and the status of the search process until the committee is ready to make its recommendation. They may not discriminate on the basis of race, sex, ethnic background, age, or physical disability against candidates, and they should be acquainted with antidiscrimination employment laws from the outset. Set forth the rules with regard to how the vote on and/or recommendation of a candidate will be accomplished.
- Present the work plan to the committee. (See Chapter 14 for details on the work plan.)

- Discuss, agree upon, and put in writing a final, detailed position specification. Construction of the position specification is an extremely important item that needs to be addressed in the early work of the committee. It will be discussed at length in a subsequent chapter.

Before the search committee begins identifying candidates, all of these matters should be addressed. It's extremely important that the rules for the working of the search committee be laid out by the chair and that these other steps be taken before the real work of the committee commences. Whether it takes one or more meetings to complete these tasks, the chair will need to be certain that they are done if a focused search is to proceed at reasonable speed.

CHAPTER 14

The Work Plan

Different time and performance priorities characterize different types of searches in the health care field. A strategic work plan will orient committee members to their roles within the search process. A search for a vice president for medical management, for instance, normally takes much less time than a search for a chair of surgery, because the latter requires more and different issues to be addressed and people to be consulted before a suitable candidate can be chosen. For example, if the chair of surgery will have to relate directly with the dean of a medical school, the dean may have to be consulted (or may be a member of the committee). The type of organization into which the chair of surgery must fit may dictate that members of the department be consulted. (See also Part III, Chapter 11.)

The work plan should be outlined in draft by the chair prior to the committee's initial meeting and then be presented at that meeting. (See Appendix 1.) The work plan and the goals it sets forth should be open to discussion, but, while welcoming constructive criticism, the chair must firmly prevent serious distortions. The most common criticism likely to arise about the work plan is that it doesn't allow for "moving quickly enough."

Developing a Work Plan

Generally, the work of a search committee can be divided into four phases:

- Developing a position specification.
- Identifying candidates.
- Interviewing candidates.
- Recommending a final candidate.

Recall that the search committee's work stops short of offering employment and negotiating compensation with the recommended candidate.

The work plan details the goals and time frame of the search. The rule of thumb here is to be realistic about time. As noted in Part I, Chapter 5, under "Selecting and Working with a Search Consultant," the typical physician-leader search takes 12 to 24 months when a search committee proceeds on its own; with the help of a firm specializing in physician-leadership search, the committee can anticipate closure within six months. Forecasts of a quicker conclusion to such a search are almost always doomed, because few committees are blessed with the strong leadership and unwavering focus (not to mention the felicity of circumstance) that a successful, short search requires.

A tight work plan has saved some foundering searches. In a 300-bed community teaching hospital located in the Philadelphia area, a search committee had been working on its own for more than two years to find a chair of surgery. It had been stymied in its attempts to identify suitable candidates and to come to closure with anyone at all. When invited to help, our first step was to lay out a detailed work plan with a demanding timetable and then to insist that everyone stick to it. This resulted in the hiring of a solid candidate less than six months later.

Time Allocations

The chair must consider each of the four phases of the upcoming search and decide how much time should be allocated for each. The sample work plan in Appendix 1 gives a general idea of appropriate allocations.

Time allocations will most likely need to be reassessed and realigned at some point, whether or not a search consultant is involved. Searches can get bogged down because of difficulty with committee meeting schedules, delays in candidate interviews, and more. But adjustment of timetables need not compromise the development of an appropriate array of candidates, as long as the chair has carefully laid the groundwork and continues to provide vigorous leadership for the committee. The chair should advise the committee that some time slippage will probably occur and ask members to suggest how to minimize it.

If there are significant time restraints—e.g., "replace the chair of medicine in six months"—the committee should use its initial meeting, in part, to consider inviting specialty search firms to make timely bids on managing all, or part of, the search. A subcommittee might be formed to quickly evaluate bids by search firms. This can easily be done within a two-week period, and a decision can be made without sacrificing any time in the process. While it entertains these bids, the committee can continue to advance the search on its own. Meanwhile, it can retain the option to wait until the point (if there is one) when the search becomes unwieldy or behind schedule before it engages outside help. Or it can wait until it reaches the specific juncture where it believes the consultant can most contribute to speeding up the process and to bringing it to a successful end—that is, when the committee feels that it cannot identify an adequate pool of candidates, or when so many candidates have been identified that outside resources are needed to sort through them in relation to the position specification.

In one case, a university hospital looking for a chair of surgery engaged a search firm to review the credentials of candidates whom the committee had identified through the "old boy network." After nine months of meeting, deliberating, and evaluating "their" candidates, committee members still could not agree on a solid prospect. The search firm's involvement was then stepped up to include the identification of new candidates from outside the "old boy network." This expansion of the candidate pool led to a successful conclusion just eight weeks later.

Member Allocations

The division of committee members' labor is the other important part of the work plan. Individuals may be enlisted to concentrate on one or more phases of the search. This allocation of responsibility should take into account the skill and the availability of each member. One member (or more—a potential subcommittee!) may be a skilled writer and could draft the position specification; others may be good interpersonal communicators (or enjoy public relations) and have the time and inclination to entertain prospective candidates who visit the area for interviews.

Assigning members to different search phases according to their strengths, interests, and availability will move the search process along more efficiently and effectively. For instance, a committee member new to the organization might be a good "match" for prospective physician-leaders of the same age. As another example, the chief of anesthesia might spend some quiet time alone with a prospective chief of surgery, elaborating on the demand for surgical services and describing the culture and personality of the organization. Keep in mind that the committee is the front-line representative of the organization; candidates will set great store by the manner in which it conducts its business and judge the opportunity being presented accordingly.

TOP DOCS

Part IV

The Candidates

CHAPTER 15

Identifying Choice Candidates

The process of identifying candidates who adequately match the position specification is the most difficult—some would say the most tedious—task in the search committee process. It is also the task in which a consultant's expertise is often most welcomed by the search committee. It involves recruitment and review of respondents to the initial recruitment efforts.

A search may be internal, external, or a combination of both. Candidates can be located through active and/or passive recruitment techniques. Active recruitment relies on aggressively accessing various informal and formal networks for candidate referrals. Passive recruitment is another name for advertising—putting the position into the market and waiting for potential candidates to respond. Overall, a recruitment effort combining passive and active methods will yield the richest pool of qualified candidates.

Internal vs. External Search

Left to their own devices, members of most search committees will probably tend to look first for candidates among physicians already on their organization's staff. However, specifications for the ideal candidate may include executive experience and accomplishments, along with clinical skills. To find such a combination internally, the committee chair and/or members might review the credentials of staff members who have been active on various hospital committees or who have held paid positions on staff—as director of medical education or director of a residency program, for instance.

Such a physician may be part of a group practice that already admits to a hospital; that group will probably be delighted at the prospect of gaining influence through the advancement of one of its members to a leadership position. A wise search committee will ponder, however, whether the elevation of an internal staff candidate might engender resentment from physicians belonging to other group practices affiliated with the hospital. Might they perceive that the choice of this new chair signals excessive hospital favor for his or her group? Will they balk if, say, the new chair of medicine demands that they do things the way the competing groups do them?

On the whole, it is usually advantageous to recruit physician-leaders from outside the organization. As competition in health care becomes ever more feverish and responsibilities more complex and challenging, recruiting from outside will become the norm. It makes more sense for a hospital to find a new physician to fill a leadership position (and, if he or she chooses, to start a new group practice) than it does to appeal to already-affiliated doctors as though it is giving anyone a competitive edge.

Active Recruitment

A common method of active recruitment is for search committee members to suggest individuals whom they, their friends, or their colleagues know might be interested. At its most constricted, this technique comprises the "old boy network." The more *au courant* search committee will expand its pool of "old boys" to include young and non-boy prospects who, although personally unknown, have distinguished themselves in impressive ways.

Indeed, there is no reason not to approach physicians known to be product line champions in their current markets, as long as the health care organization has the wherewithal to attract and retain these "top" top docs. They can benefit a hospital directly. Aiming for the best and the brightest is worth the effort. You can identify "clinical leaders" in a specific specialty by a few well-placed calls to key educators in major medical schools throughout the country. Six calls could get you at least 12 names.

A few strategic phone calls to key officers at professional associations will also activate the recruitment grapevine. Don't overlook the annual meetings of professional associations as a way to advertise your position and as a forum to meet with prospective candidates. The American Society of Anesthesiologists does a noteworthy job of encouraging and assisting with recruitment activities of its members at its annual convention. Other associations also have workable arrangements.

Although active recruitment can identify candidates fairly quickly, it demands a significant commitment of time from search committee members and runs the risk of resulting in a small, rather shallow candidate pool. A wider group of prospects can be reached through passive recruitment.

Passive Recruitment

The major passive recruitment tactic is advertising in trade or association publications, major newspapers, and medical journals. A substantial response to such advertising is guaranteed—and a lot of it will come from ill-suited candidates. While sometimes successful, the mountain of responses from advertising presents an unmanageable task to most committees. Few of these responses are thoroughly reviewed.

Some hospitals in remote, rural areas have received publicity in recent years for offering bounties, usually to local citizens and medical staff members who suggest the names of staff doctors to be recruited. This is a combined active and passive approach. The bounty is paid when the search committee recommends a suggested candidate for hire, and it may be supplemented at certain stages during the new physician's first few years of service. But recruitment of physician-leaders is likely to proceed more sedately, even in these hospitals. By the time they have reached the point in their careers where they might be considered for a leadership position, physicians (and their high-level peers on the committees searching for them) are likely to find bounties or other premium payments a distasteful approach to recruitment.

CHAPTER 16

Selecting the Choicest Candidates

When it comes to recruiting a physician-leader, it is likely that the search committee will know a fair amount about the candidates (or at least their reputations) before they are directly approached. This is certainly true if a search consultant is involved in identifying appropriate prospects. It is the job of either that consultant or, absent outside help, of the chair to ask candidates for their "paper," or curriculum vitae (CV).

Sometimes, candidates, reluctant to throw their hats in the ring formally, will hesitate to send their CVs. In these cases, learn as much as possible by talking directly with the candidate (taking care not to scare the physician off) and independently developing a brief candidate background sketch. This can be supplemented by confidential comments from others who have known or worked with the candidate. From this information, determine whether to pursue a candidate. It is amazing how many initially reluctant candidates will succumb to the flattery of being courted by a search committee.

It is the responsibility of the search committee to review the "paper" on each prospect, looking for overall fit with the position specification. Internal candidates should be screened exactly as those from outside are screened. It's usually a waste of the committee's time to meet with a candidate solely on the basis of the CV, however. The "paper" needs to be supplemented with telephone conversations, at least, so that the search committee can get some idea of the potential match between the prospect and the position specification.

Matching Paper to Spec

The job of matching candidates' CVs and other evidence with the position spec is not as easy as it sounds. The search committee's review of each candidate's background must also include a comprehensive analysis of the physician's career, professional career path, accomplishments, and scope of responsibility. Usually only direct personal contact with candidates (best done before bringing them before the committee) can secure this information.

This time-consuming step causes many search committees to stumble. It can be tedious and frustrating, and knowledgeable committees are often happy to turn the hours of telephone tag, detailed conversations, and face-to-face meetings over to a search consultant. In any case, a search's success is strongly linked to this stage's thoroughness in exploring candidates' backgrounds and accomplishments.

Screening and Selecting

Some applicants will be disqualified out of hand because their academic backgrounds, experience, or achievements are clearly inadequate. Others will more closely meet the spec's demands, although not in all areas. A few may be weak in just one area. Rarely does a candidate meet the spec absolutely.

Obviously, those who come closest will constitute the first tier of candidates to be personally contacted by the committee chair or cochair. There should be three to five candidates, agreed upon by vote of the entire committee. A second tier of candidates can be formed in case no one in the first tier pans out.

Consider, however, that the second tier of candidates will always be looked upon as being "second best." Regardless of how diligent the committee may be in not describing these candidates as inferior to the first group, they may be perceived as less than adequate. Recognizing how language influences opinion is one way of managing around this dilemma. Avoid calling the second group "back-up candidates" or "the second tier" in speech, writing, or even thought. Furthermore, the chair can ask the committee to agree that the search will focus on a few candidates at a time. This will help to avoid the notion that some candidates are inferior to others.

CHAPTER 17

Managing the Candidates

Up to this point, the search committee may have indulged in a bit of internecine sniping. But the handling of candidates who qualify for the open leadership position can turn those isolated, random shots into a hail of bullets. Improperly managed, this aspect of the search committee process can make a hospital seem like the "O.K. Corral."

There will have been no specific focus to any earlier disagreements, even rancorous ones, regarding the role that the new physician-leader will play in the organization. Once flesh-and-blood candidates enter the picture, a clearer, more intense spotlight will shine on certain issues. For instance, there might be strong opinions about the effect a new chief of cardiology will have on existing staff internists and their referral patterns. Candidates' responses to some committee members' questions might be read in various ways, providing a platform from which such an issue, already the source of friction, may be more vehemently debated. Worse, members of search committees have been known to bait candidates with certain questions in an effort to get answers that will work to those members' advantage.

Limited Exposure

As candidate management comes to the fore, one or two committee members should be assigned to respond to prospects' queries and to solicit needed information from them. These liaisons should also be responsible for keeping candidates as fully informed as possible throughout the search. This will help to maintain consistency, which is crucial to the handling of candidates during a successful physician-leader search.

Restricting candidates' access to search committee members (and vice versa) also helps to ensure consistency. The fewer people they talk to, the less likely candidates are to get a muddled notion of the available opportunity. If a search consultant is involved, he or she becomes the conduit of all information flowing between the candidate and the committee, further enhancing consistency.

The time to enlarge serious candidates' exposure is the interview phase. This requires considerable logistical legerdemain. It also cries out for more personal sensitivity than it often gets.

Managing the Interview Process

The candidate interview phase can be handled a number of ways, depending on a particular search committee's agreed-upon preferences and/or the availability of committee members. It is important that interviews be carefully scheduled, not only in respect of the value of physicians' time, but also to avoid leaving candidates with unstructured, wasted hours.

A subcommittee of one or more members might conduct one- to two-hour preliminary interviews with candidates as a means of further screening them for desired background, accomplishments, attitude, etc. Those who "pass" would advance to extensive interviews with the entire committee.

Alternatively, each candidate might be interviewed by the search committee as a whole, or by individual members, in scheduled, one-hour, back-to-back sessions. Group interviews (i.e., interviews conducted by some or all members of the committee at the same time) are most easily managed in conjunction with a luncheon or a committee dinner that generally lasts for two or more hours.

Taken one at a time, it is possible for the committee to interview all available candidates in one day *if* each committee member can schedule an extended outlay of time during the same day. The higher the volume of candidates to be seen in one day, the greater the need for controlled coordination of schedules by the chair. Candidates who pass one another in the hall or are seated side by side to wait for an interview can be embarrassed or annoyed. In addition, the confidentiality concerns of candidates need to be taken into account when structuring interviews. For instance, a well-known candidate may be wary of being noticed and may forgo a hospital tour or ask to be interviewed after hours.

The Personal Touch

In any case, candidates should be managed with careful consideration throughout the interview process, which, after all, sows the seeds for a future working relationship. Perhaps because they are unaware (or do not acknowledge) that little things mean a lot in relationships, physician-leader search committees often mishandle this phase, overlooking simple steps that candidates value. For example, candidates should be formally greeted by the chair when they arrive for their interviews and then be given a tour of the facility. This allows the candidate to relax a bit, to gather more information prior to interviews, and to form impressions that he or she may want to investigate further during interviews.

Candidates should be escorted throughout their visits, with introductions to each interviewer made in a pleasant, businesslike manner. Some search committee procedures call for entertaining candidates in the evening. They may also entail informal meetings with spouses; these are best conducted over dinner. (See Appendix 6, "Candidate Interview Agenda.")

Debriefing the Candidates

One of the most important aspects of candidate management is the debriefing that should closely follow the round of meetings, meals, tours, etc. Soliciting summary comments and reactions from the candidate at the end of the day is an excellent tool for gauging his or her level of continued interest in the position. Additionally, candidate concerns should be seriously evaluated and answered quickly in order to maintain the candidate's interest. The chair, cochair, and/or the search consultant can all play useful roles in this process.

One candidate for a chief of pathology position ended his day of interviews disconsolately, having "heard" repeatedly how important it was for the successful applicant to be available "as soon as possible." Knowing that his current contract committed him to 90 day's notice and that a critical research project demanded his presence during that time, he felt his chances for landing the position were nonexistent. He was open about his concern during his debriefing at the end of that day. As a result, the committee was able to clarify for him that "as soon as possible" meant 60 to 90 days—and that additional time was not out of the question. The candidate and the committee, back in synch, eventually came to closure.

Committee members or the consultant, acting as liaison to candidates, are responsible for contacting interviewees for debriefing. Promptness is paramount. Laggard liaison not only leaves a poor impression of the organization, but also allows a time lapse that can dull memory and perceptions. And it drags out the search committee process.

In debriefing candidates, be sure to inquire about:

- The candidate's level of interest in the position and whether it has changed.
- Any significant candidate concerns about the position or about continuing to pursue it.
- Any additional information the candidate might need to evaluate the opportunity.
- People with whom the candidate might want to meet in subsequent interviews.
- The spouse's level of interest in the position and relocation (if appropriate); the relocation discussion might also cover special arrangements for locating new employment for the spouse.

Finally, the debriefer must describe to the candidate the next steps and the timing of the process.

Candidates' debriefing comments should be summarized and shared with the committee in its next meeting. If a search consultant is involved, these summaries can be put in writing for the record, for further review by the chair, and for delivery to all committee members prior to the next meeting.

Chapter 18

Evaluating the Candidates

Prompt action by the search committee as a whole is essential in ensuring that each candidate's in-person "performance" is evaluated fairly and that the search committee process keeps moving apace. Consequently, candidates aren't the only ones who should be debriefed. The full committee should hold a debriefing session as soon as possible after a day of interviews—ideally at the end of that same day.

Members who have met individually with candidates should debrief committee colleagues in a group meeting as soon as possible—again, preferably on the same day. Their comments regarding interviewees' personal and professional presentations, qualifications, motivations, and other factors should be carefully recorded in the minutes. A Candidate Evaluation Form tailored for the specific position may also be used to expedite this process. (See Appendix 7.)

If a consultant is participating in the search, he or she can debrief both the search committee and the candidate following interviews. If either party expresses confusion or concern, the consultant should work as a mediator to resolve any problems or perceptions. In this role, the consultant is able to keep candidates uniformly advised about the organization and the open position, as well as to provide them all with the same procedural instructions.

Evaluation Process Management

It's also a good idea for someone on the committee, preferably the chair or the cochair, to record committee members' comments on each candidate's fit suitability for the position. These notes will prove to be valuable when candidates are further discussed by the committee with an eye toward return interviews.

It helps in managing candidates through the process if the note-taker indicates who made what comments about each candidate. For instance, one member of the committee may have had a problem with a candidate's response to a specific question. This is worth following up in committee discussions about the candidate, as well as with the candidate during a second round of interviews. Notes might also flag for the chair any committee members whose initial reactions to a candidate were generally positive, but whose comments after a second round of interviews were markedly, and specifically, more critical.

A thorough and prompt debriefing of the search committee is particularly important when a number of candidates are being considered, for candidates tend to blend together in members' minds as time passes. A review of notes taken in the debriefing session will serve as a concrete reminder of each candidate's strengths and weaknesses.

It is the role of the chair (or the chair's designated liaison) to promptly advise any candidates who have been eliminated from competition as a result of their first round of interviews with the committee. This can be done in a telephone discussion followed up by a thank-you note from the chair of the search committee. If the phone call yields any useful candidate feedback, the committee representative should record it and share it with the full search committee at its next formal session.

Final Rounds

Candidates may go through two or three more interviews with the search committee, each time progressing in their understanding of the position and the organization, as well as refining their areas of concern. As in the first interview, candidate debriefings continue to be extremely important. Debriefings should be conducted after each encounter with the candidate, as in round one.

Search committee debriefings also remain on the agenda. The search committee will refine and refocus its concerns, questions, and observations about a candidate through each round of interviews. The strongest foundation for this is proper debriefing. Methodical recording of concerns and comments should also continue.

Referencing the Candidates

Formal referencing activities can begin after a candidate's first round of interviews, as long as there seems to be committee consensus that the candidate deserves serious consideration.

Preliminary Referencing

There are different levels of referencing activity. Preliminary referencing includes verification of dates of education, employment, medical licensing, and board certification. With the exception of dates of employment, all other information can be easily acquired without disrupting the candidate's current employment relationship. (See Appendix 8, "Physician Credential Check.") Many educational institutions and licensing and accrediting bodies will not release information without a candidate's written permission. The medical staff executive secretary or a secretary assigned to support the work of the search committee could be assigned to obtain this release from the candidate.

The search committee should make it a point to ensure that the preliminary referencing data are gathered before a candidate's second visit. This will ensure that the need for this information will not get lost in the shuffle. Do not allow a candidate to move through the search committee process without some general verification of his or her background, education, and employment, at the very least. It is also a good idea to attach the results of the referencing to the file of information gathered on the candidate so that it is prominently displayed for the chairman to evaluate prior to each new step.

Queries to the National Practitioner Data Bank, which records unfavorable actions taken against physicians, might also be appropriate before embarking on a second round of interviews with any candidate. This can be done only with the candidate's approval.

Referencing Chats

Referencing conversations with peers, subordinates, and superiors of the prospective candidate are usually undertaken when both committee and candidate show serious interest in each other. This is another delicate step, because inappropriate contacts with prospective references could jeopardize the candidate's current employment relationship. It is extremely important that informal referencing not be initiated by members of the committee without the knowledge and approval of the candidate.

In spite of repeated cautions against informal referencing, the CEO of a hospital considering a candidate for a chief of anesthesia position phoned an affiliated hospital in the town where the candidate for the position lived, purportedly to "check out" the candidate casually before proceeding to the next level of interviews. The candidate was in the final stages of renegotiating his current contract when word of the call got back to his department chief. Needless to say, this did not exactly grease his contract negotiations, nor did it improve his prospects for a long-term relationship with his current chief in his view. The candidate thus withdrew his candidacy for the chief of anesthesia position and filed a lawsuit against the recruiting institution. The suit was settled before going to trial. In this case, the hospital CEO's inappropriate actions cost the institution tangibly, in attorneys' fees and settlement expenses, and possibly intangibly, in terms of industry approbation.

Usually, it is the candidate who provides a list of references for the committee to contact. It is advisable for the committee to stay attuned to names and relationships that candidates cite in the course of interviews. These individuals, who may not have been offered by the candidate, are fair game for a reference list.

The chair of the committee or the committee's candidate liaison is responsible for receiving a candidate's suggested reference list and for proposing additional names to the candidate. Candidate hesitancy about including these other names needs to be probed. Such reluctance might arise from concern about jeopardizing the current employment relationship, of course. But it could also be that the candidate is trying to evade questions about poor performance or negative events in his or her past. In the end, however, it is extremely important to remember that referencing should not be done without the candidate's approval.

Referencing Techniques

A single individual or a small group should be given the task of checking references. This maintains consistency in the areas of questioning, style, and presentation. One person—a skilled listener and analyst—doing all of the referencing can pick up on subtle hints of dissatisfaction or concern and then seek expansion on them in subsequent conversations or by talking again with other references. When several individuals are involved in the referencing process, this ability may be compromised or lost.

Referencing conversations are usually confidential and should be so recorded and maintained. Taking notes during a telephone conversation and reducing them to a confidential summary is generally sufficient. (See Appendix 9, "Sample Reference Report.") The summary should identify the candidate; the date of the reference; the person giving the reference; and, briefly, that person's relationship with the candidate. Although the reference checker will know what is said, and the chair of the search committee might have access to the notes, details of these conversations should not be shared with the committee as a whole. The chair should summarize key comments for the committee without attributing them to any particular reference.

What if these referencing chats turn up some concerns about a candidate? Naturally, they should be explored with other references, whether already on record or not, and possibly with additional references that the candidate might be asked to provide. Any questions, weaknesses, poor relationships, etc. should be thoroughly aired with references, and sometimes with the candidate as well, before proceeding to the next level of interviews. An attentive referencer will differentiate between areas that simply need improvement and those of real concern. The former can be shared with the search committee and followed up in subsequent candidate interviews, but they do not require the extensive investigation warranted by real "red flags."

CHAPTER 19

Recommending the Choicest of the Choice

It is the search committee's job to recommend a final candidate to the health care organization's CEO or governing board. Whether this job is gut-wrenching and tumultuous, or calm and businesslike, has a great deal to do with all the steps that have come before it. In this, the crisis phase of the search committee's life story, the groundwork and the leadership provided by the chair will play a key role.

A committee searching for a chief of physiatry was about to recommend the appointment of an internal candidate for the position. This decision came after much discussion within the committee on the qualifications of the internal candidate, but also at a time when several stronger, external candidates had withdrawn. The committee was about to recommend the appointment of the internal candidate when the CEO got involved. Having heard of the debate from the administration's representative on the committee, the CEO advised the search chair in no uncertain terms that the internal candidate was unacceptable and that he would not recommend appointment by the hospital's board.

Fortunately, an actual vote had not yet been taken, so the chair was able to save face for himself and the committee. He told the committee that the internal candidate did not hew to the agreed-upon position specification and then offered two choices. First, the committee could rewrite the position specification to take into account the internal candidate's levels of experience and capability, which were well below those put forth in the original spec. While allowing the internal candidate to qualify fully for the position, this approach would also open up the job to a larger field of candidates in the market who had not previously been considered. The second option was for the committee to stick to the original spec and advise the internal candidate that his qualifications were not satisfactory. The committee chose the latter step.

Gaining Consensus

Even the most arduous labor by the chair cannot always produce quick, unanimous approval of a single candidate. Perhaps half of top doc search committees unanimously endorse a candidate on the first vote. Some bickering usually accompanies the committee's final selection process. It can escalate unpleasantly, but, if the search committee has been consistently oriented toward consensus, more quiet discussion is likely to dominate. In such an atmosphere, the chair has a better chance of coaxing unanimity from an initial majority vote.

The chair may try a review of the candidates interviewed to date to determine whether a consensus can be gained for any of them without the process of a formal vote. This typically is done after three to five candidates have been interviewed. By straw votes that test the sentiment of the committee toward candidates, the chair can fairly predict the candidate most likely to emerge as the final choice.

The search consultant can contribute immeasurably by formally comparing each candidate to the position specification and by presenting this comparison to the committee as a stimulus to conversation. Such a presentation can also help to reaffirm the direction of the committee, which may have become a bit hazy in the interviewing and referencing stages. Keeping the committee focused is an ongoing imperative, of course, but this is a point where it comes into special play. If the process has not produced candidates who meet the position specification, or if the specification itself is faulty, failing to specifically and accurately translate the goals of the hospital and the committee into a description of the best-qualified candidate, a reassessment is absolutely necessary before further work is done.

If in-fighting on the committee has made consensus impossible, it is not unprecedented for an institution to disband the committee and form a new one. A hospital that takes this drastic step needs to add to the new committee members who will re-energize it, people who can stave off disruption.

However, disbanding the committee and replacing the chair are not especially desirable options. They present serious, long-term problems for the institution and for its relationships with key physicians. Persevering through the process and attempting to manage it may sometimes seem harder, but it is preferable. One way of breaking a disruptive deadlock is to appoint new members to the committee as the process unfolds. Although this technique has proved to be the most successful approach to total impasse, it certainly brings on headaches of its own.

The chair may try "shuttle diplomacy" outside formal meetings to move members of the committee toward a consensus. Too heavy-handed an approach can backfire, however, painfully fracturing the committee process. It is advisable for the chair to use the position specification that the committee has approved as a point of reference when drawing finer comparisons on some candidates.

Frequently, writing down how each candidate under consideration stacks up against the major specifications for the position helps to highlight strengths and weaknesses in the backgrounds of various candidates. (Appendix 10 contains an example of such a written comparison.) Having to commit these judgments to writing tends to focus the thoughts of committee members on precisely what they had set out to achieve at the outset of the search process.

In discussing comments made by references, a given candidate may become more attractive to the committee, which can swing the vote toward a major consensus. The search consultant can help at this point; he or she will know if a number of people recommended a candidate early in the process and/or if the same candidate's name often comes up in the market during searches for prospective candidates.

For all the mention of speeding up top doc searches, there are occasions when the chair can use delay to his or her advantage. Wearing down members of the committee by dragging out the process is a technique that numerous search committee chairs have employed to get consensus. It's a "wait and hurry up," filibustering process, although it should never assume the noisy proportions of a congressional maneuver.

If the months have dragged on, with search committee meeting after boring meeting punctuated by moments of incivility and wounded feelings, and only the barest majority of members firmly support a single, preferred candidate, a major rethinking of the process is required. Sometimes it is best to disband the committee and start over again. Injection of new members to the committee might be helpful as well as possibly the appointment of a new chairman. All the above have been tried with varying degrees of success. In general, however, it's better to keep the committee together, attempt to reinvigorate it by focusing attention on those members of the committee who don't seem to be pulling in the direction of the others.

It is at this point that a search consultant can frequently be of enormous help. An outside influence, an "expert" stepping back from the process, can realistically advise a committee on how to get going again. Most times, it doesn't take a complete restart, just a reexamination of candidates who have already passed through the committee and/or a redefinition of the requirements for the position. Sometimes a more thorough, more deliberate, and more organized approach to the market will produce additional candidates in a very short period.

It may be that adjusting items such as compensation, reporting relationship, or organizational structure—things that will seem minor in retrospect—is all that is required to get the process moving again. But, whether the agent is a search consultant brought in from the outside, a new chair, or a cochair, the committee must take a fresh direction, or it will surely wither and die.

Making the Choice: Public Ballot

The advantage of a public ballot, of course, is that it tells the chair who the supporters of each candidate are, so that the chair can target non-supporters for whatever persuasion is necessary. A straw vote taken prior to the "official" vote will give the chair an early sense of the standing of particular candidates.

Another advantage of the public ballot is its influence on fence-sitters. Often, those who are undecided about a candidate will hesitate to say so in a public forum. Alternatively, they may be more reluctant to publicly oppose a candidate than to go along with the majority.

The danger in a public ballot is that, having made their positions clear, some people may refuse to reconsider in the interest of consensus. If they set their feet, it may be quite difficult to get them to change their votes in subsequent balloting.

Making the Choice: Secret Ballot

Unless the chair has a clear indication of unanimous support for a candidate, the secret ballot is probably the best approach to concluding the process. Committee members who may not conversationally support a particular candidate for fear of alienating their peers may very well vote for that candidate on a secret ballot. However, the reverse is also true: someone who did not, in discussions, oppose a candidate to avoid alienating a peer on the committee may vote against that candidate on a secret ballot.

The decision to move ahead with a public or a secret ballot is sometimes a very tough one for a chair. The rule of thumb generally is, "If you don't feel you can reasonably predict the outcome of the ballot, use a secret ballot." The chairman must then work (albeit in a more general way than if everyone's vote were known) to influence a change in the vote for a subsequent secret balloting.

It's ugly, but it has to be said: Some search committee chairs have been known to misstate the results of a secret ballot, especially when *they* collect the votes.

Making the Choice: No Ballot At All

Although by far the exceptional approach, some chairs reserve the right to make the selection of a candidate without an actual vote of the search committee. This can only be done in that rare circumstance in which the chair is a uniquely strong individual, not only in personality but also politically, in the medical staff hierarchy. If a chair wants to proceed this way, he or she must, at the outset of the committee process, make a strong statement as to how the recommendation of the candidate will be made. Otherwise, committee anarchy could result. Overall, this is not a recommended approach.

TOP DOCS

Part V

The Money and More

Chapter 20

Structuring a Compensation Package

The actual compensation arrangement that is appropriate for any given institution or physician-leader is not a boilerplate matter. The right form depends on the type of hospital, the institutional culture, and the objectives of the organization in acquiring the talents of a particular physician-leader. What is more important than the form the compensation arrangement takes is its fairness and reasonableness in the eyes of both the physician and the organization, and its relationship to the realities of the marketplace.

The Market Effect

Assessing the market for a particular physician-leader position involves ferreting out reference material about compensation ranges from a variety of sources—many of them hidden. When unearthed, many sources may communicate in torturous jargon, if they are willing to share information at all. Added to these concerns is the difficulty of meaningfully comparing any available data with the open position. The scope and responsibilities of positions, even in similar markets, can vary widely.

The following published physician compensation surveys can be useful in bracketing a market range for a physician leadership position.

- American Association of Medical Colleges (AAMC)—Faculty Survey.
- Medical Group Management Association (MGMA)—Physician Compensation and Production Survey.
- Wm. Mercer—Survey of Total Compensation of U.S. Physician Employees.
- Ernst and Young—Physician Compensation and Productivity Survey.
- Hay Group—Physician Total Compensation Survey.

Some "benchmark" physician-leader positions have come to be similarly defined by a great many institutions, however. One is vice president for medical management. From the early 1980s, while the traditional medical director position was turning into this position in most hospitals, there was much compensation variability in the market. It was difficult to establish a realistic compensation range, because job responsibilities were generally ill-defined. Frequently, compensation for the position was driven by the specialty of the physician who filled it. A surgeon, for instance, might start at a higher base compensation rate as a vice president for medical management than would a pediatrician. As the job responsibilities for this position became better defined, however, a market range of compensation that allowed more predictability evolved. In 1999, a typical vice president for medical management in a 350- to 450-bed community teaching hospital earns in the range of $225,000 to $275,000, regardless of his or her specialty.*

As other physician-leadership positions assume clearer definition in the years to come, their compensation ranges will also settle in. Until then, the best that a health care organization can do in targeting the appropriate range for any physician-leader, especially if his or her primary responsibilities are clinical, is to use whatever published information is available and to survey the local market for compensation data on similar positions. (See Appendix 11, "Physician Leadership Compensation Ranges." for a sample of such a survey.) That base of information can be expanded as current compensation arrangements of various candidates considered for an open position are added.

With the health care industry going through such rapid changes, the issue of physician compensation is likely to be a subject of fervent debate for a number of years. More benchmark physician-leadership positions will probably develop. Meanwhile, a hiring organization can seldom go wrong with a thorough survey of similar positions in its local market to determine an appropriate range of compensation. The time to conduct such a survey is, of course, before candidates enter the picture.

Whatever the amount involved, the compensation package for a physician-leadership candidate encompasses four major items:

- Cash compensation.
- Non-cash compensation.
- Benefits and perquisites.
- Contractual arrangements.

Cash Compensation: Salary

Cash compensation for physician-leadership candidates is usually distributed in a way that plays off one of three general themes: salary, administrative stipend/clinical income, or a faculty practice plan arrangement. Variable compensation in the form of bonuses and incentive compensation are becoming more frequent components of the compensation package for physician-leaders.

---

* Longshore, G. "An Emerging Leadership Position." *Physician Executive* 22(9):18-22, Sept. 1996.

Salaried compensation is typical of physician-leadership positions in which a significant portion of time is allocated to administrative, supervisory, and teaching (AS&T) activities. When AS&T responsibilities, rather than hands-on clinical responsibilities, dominate the job, most (if not all) cash compensation is provided in the form of salary. Positions to which this would commonly apply include vice president for medical affairs, director of quality assurance and utilization review, director of residency training, and director of medical education.

Along with a base salary for such positions, it is not unusual to find a bonus or other additional incentive compensation. This harks back to the perception that these positions are, by and large, more administrative than clinical in the overall table of hospital organization. If the position has broad responsibilities touching on various clinical programs throughout the organization (as a vice president for medical management might), a bonus or other form of incentive compensation will probably be offered. It will be tied to both profitability and the physician-leader's achievement of individual objectives.

When hospital-based physicians (in emergency medicine, anesthesia, pathology, and radiology) are salaried, variable compensation is added to their compensation packages. This variable compensation is commonly linked to the performance of the relevant clinical department. For instance, an emergency medicine physician might find his or her bonus contingent on a specific increase in the number of emergency department visits and/or a reduction in wait time for emergency department patients.

Cash Compensation: Administrative Stipend/Clinical Income

Compensation for positions that entail more direct clinical activity and accountability and fewer AS&T responsibilities popularly combines an administrative stipend and a share in, or retention of, all clinical income produced by the physician-leader. The income generated by the physician's department may also be factored into the latter part of this equation. For instance, a chief of obstetrics and gynecology in a community teaching hospital might be given an administrative stipend of $50,000 a year for spending up to 15 hours a week in AS&T activities, plus all of the income generated from his or her clinical activities.

In some cases, however, a hospital will strike a deal featuring a cap on clinical income. Beyond that amount, the hospital shares clinical revenues with the physician.

Administrative stipend/clinical income arrangements may also be structured with a revenue threshold; that is, the physician must first generate a certain amount of income before he or she can begin to share in amounts that exceed the threshold. The theory here is that the hospital intends to recover the cost of employing this physician before allowing the physician to share in revenue generated.

Cash Compensation: Faculty Practice Plan Arrangements

Details of faculty practice plan arrangements vary widely in form and substance. However, most are similar in their major elements. One of these is a set "salary" that the physician draws during the year. Clinical income generated by the physician and by others in the department is pooled, and, after direct and indirect expenses are subtracted, the remainder is distributed among all the physicians who generated the income according to a formula. Outside income from royalties, honoraria, visiting professorship salaries, etc. are generally considered in these computations, although they may or may not be included when the formula is applied to determining final compensation. In the end, a department's net income is often allocated to its physicians on the basis of seniority and/or rank.

Non-Cash Compensation

Items frequently not initially considered but customarily included in the compensation package for a clinical leader include the value of office space, support staff, equipment, practice management services, billing services, and malpractice insurance. These items not only need to be discussed as part of the overall offering prior to interviewing candidates, but also should be factored into the value of the total compensation proposed for the chosen candidate.

The Internal Revenue Service and the Office of the Inspector General (OIG) are showing serious interest in applying the test of "reasonableness of compensation" for physician-leaders. Stories of "magnet doctors" recruited and paid exorbitant salaries have already attracted the OIG's attention. Both cash and the value of non-cash compensation will be subject to scrutiny. In this regard, market-based compensation data from published sources and from individual hospital/search committee surveys will help to protect the hospital by providing solid evidence of local compensation practices.

Benefits

The value of benefits and perks should also be considered as part of the overall cost of recruiting and engaging a new physician-leader. Benefits commonly provided for full time, hospital-based physicians include:

- Payment of malpractice insurance premiums (usually limited to $1–3 million coverage).
- Payment of health insurance premiums (a contribution for family coverage, may be required).
- Payment of life insurance premiums (coverage equaling, on average, two times base salary).
- Payment of short-term and long-term disability insurance premiums.
- A pension plan (physician must contribute, however).
- Four weeks of vacation for first five years of service.

- Ten holidays, three personal days, and 11 sick days per year.
- Annual salary review.
- Payment of cost of relevant professional books, publications, reprint costs, and dues; a benefit that may be:
  - ➢ Provided for chairs and division heads only.
  - ➢ Allocated as a fixed dollar amount annually (generally $1,000 to $2,000) that may be supplemented by the department chief.
  - ➢ Individually negotiated between faculty members and hospital or department chiefs.
- Tuition reimbursement.
- Some reimbursement for special equipment. (A fixed dollar amount is usually not allocated, but if special equipment needs are not met through the capital budgeting process, payment may be individually negotiated by the physician with the hospital, the faculty practice plan, and/or the department chief.)
- Reimbursement for hospital-related business travel expenses.
- Moving expenses (a standard benefit for all faculty, for department chairs only, or as an individually negotiated benefit).
- Working space/secretary.

Perquisites

Perquisites are not standardized for physician-leaders; they vary widely. Even within a local market, there is no basic set of perquisites commonly included in a compensation package. Some popular perquisites are cited below, but the list is by no means exhaustive:

- Payment of professional dues.
- An automobile; car expenses may also be included.
- Payment of country club membership fees.
- Annual physical exam.
- Dining club membership fees.
- Costs of spouse traveling with the physician on business.
- Financial/tax counseling fees.
- Health club membership fees.
- Arrangements for personal loans at favorable rates.
- Costs of first-class business travel.

- Tuition reimbursement.
- Legal counseling fees.
- Car phone.

Contractual Arrangements

The typical contract term for a new physician-leader is two to three years. One-year, renewable contracts are the norm thereafter.

Today, contract clauses mandating that medical staff privileges end if employment ends are much more common for physician-leaders than ever before. The trend toward these "co-terminus clauses" appears to be growing in hospital-based physician specialties, such as anesthesia, pathology, radiology, and emergency medicine.

Restrictive covenants are also increasingly found in physician-leader contracts. This is because hospitals usually incur significant up-front expenses to establish their new physicians in clinical practice. Thus, they prefer to keep the new leaders in place. Rather than risking their departure at the end of the initial contract to set up practice with a competing hospital, hospitals add restrictive covenants, also known as noncompete clauses. Such clauses need to be reasonable in order to be enforceable. Legal counsel is required to help in developing the contract.

Chapter 21

Negotiating a Compensation Package

Along with market-based information about comparable compensation arrangements or similar positions locally, an analysis of the revenue that will be generated and the expenses that will be incurred by the candidate's clinical activity is necessary before negotiating a package. Appendix 12 contains a sample of this kind of analysis. This example portrays the income from clinical activity that is projected for a chief of anesthesia, plus the expenses expected in order to generate that activity. Utilizing this approach gives a hospital a better idea of what it can anticipate in terms of an overage (profit), thereby establishing the degree of flexibility that will be possible when the time comes to negotiate compensation.

Negotiating a contract with a preferred candidate for a physician-leadership position is sometimes as tricky as conducting the search itself. Once a candidate is under serious consideration by the search committee and closure seems distinctly possible, preliminary contract conversations should be held with the candidate and the hospital's administrative representative. The major points of the proposed compensation arrangement should be presented in outline form to the candidate of choice in a letter of intent (see Appendix 13). This letter not only indicates the search committee's level of interest in the candidate, but also identifies the chief items in the compensation package so that additional items are not, at a subsequent date, inserted into the arrangement. This is not, in my view, the point at which legal counsel should be invited by the hospital to become directly involved in constructing a "contract." That intervention should await the hammering out of an agreement between hospital and candidate on the main features of the compensation arrangement. Only after completion of a letter of intent that is acceptable to both parties should counsel develop the actual contract. Too many potential couplings of candidates and institutions have been derailed by attorneys who knew very little about physician compensation and contracting and interceded before they were really needed. When this happens, all the work of the search committee has been in vain.

Negotiating a compensation package that everyone feels is fair is an art. A "win-win" attitude on the part of both parties will ease the tensions around the negotiating sessions and usually make for a better outcome.

The use of agents by professional athletes in negotiating their contracts usually works well because the athlete and the team owner are kept apart by a "mediator" or agent. The athlete and the owner don't meet until the deal is ready to be signed. There is a lesson to be learned here in developing a deal with a physician-leader. Whether a search consultant or some other party in whom the candidate has developed trust, a mediator can effectively soften positions on both sides through the use of "shuttle diplomacy" before allowing the two parties to face off.

A candidate for a chief of perinatology position in a 500-bed community hospital knew the hospital's chief of neonatology, having gone through the same pediatric residency program. When it came time to negotiate the contract with the chief of perinatology, the neonatologist/friend was very helpful to the hospital's administration not only in identifying the candidate's key issues, but also in making the hospital more aware of compensation arrangements, equipment, and other practice supports provided in competing institutions.

Obviously, if a search consultant is supporting the search activity, he or she will be the mediator in the negotiating process.

The principle to remember in negotiating is "keep the parties apart until the deal is ready to be signed." A corollary to that is "keep the attorneys out of it as long as possible."

CHAPTER 22

Costs of the Search

The committee chair and the hospital CEO will have developed a budget for the search effort before the committee members are even named. The major expense categories to consider are:

- Candidate contact expenses.
- Candidate interview expenses.
- Professional fees.
- Miscellaneous expenses.

These expenses will vary with the number of candidates contacted, the number of candidates interviewed (and the number of times they are interviewed), and the geographic scope of the search and the distance traveled by the candidates.

Sample Budget: Search for Chairman of Radiology

Candidate Contact Expenses	
Advertising (e.g., *New England Journal of Medicine,* and two other professional journals) and Internet postings	$2,000
Promotional materials (probably already available through Public Relations Department)	N/C
Letters/postage (500 letters @ $.75)	325
Telephone	1,000

*Note: not factored here are labor expenses of secretarial and professional staff).

Candidate Interview Expenses—Initial Interviews

Round-trip airfare from Chicago to East or West Coast (3 candidates @ $600 each)	$1,800
Lodging, candidate only (3 candidates)	600
Taxi/car rental	200
Meals	300

Candidate Interview Expenses—Second Round of Interviews

Round-trip airfare (2 candidates and spouse—and kids?)	$2,400
Lodging	600
Taxi/car rental	300
Meals	400

Fees

Search consultant	$60,000-75,000
Attorney	4,000-6,000
Other expenses	
Moving expenses	8,000-10,000
Temporary living expenses (30 - 90 days)	5,000-7,500
Swing loan (interest expense 90-180 days)	2,000

The budget should allow for flexibility, but its limits should be understood and respected under the leadership of the chair.

Using a consultant to undertake a full search might entail a fee ranging from 30-35 percent of the successful candidate's first year's compensation. If the committee elects to do some of the search tasks on its own, employing the consulting firm only for certain activities (identifying candidates, for example), it is customary to make an hourly time-plus-expenses arrangement with the consultant. The consulting firm will then bill the committee at an hourly rate, usually ranging from $150 to $250, for the time the consultant actually spends on the project. Discounts can usually be negotiated for either arrangement, especially if the consulting firm wants your repeat business or has already established a relationship with you.

Most search firms charge clients for all out-of-pocket, search-related costs, such as telephone, travel, meals, lodging, and other expenses associated with accessing and interviewing candidates. They should do so at cost; beware of firms that mark up out-of-pocket charges. These expenses can range from 10 to 20 percent of the search fee, depending on the geographic focus of the search activity. Determine at the outset of the assignment how you want the consulting firm to itemize and document these expenses so that future questions of billing impropriety can be avoided.

TOP DOCS

Part VI

Epilog

PART VI: EPILOG

Trends and Prospects for Top Doc Searches

On January 1, 1992, Medicare's physician payment reform plan, known as the Resource-Based Relative Value Scale (RBRVS), was implemented. So radical was this change that Pete Stark, Chairman of the House Ways and Means Health Subcommittee, joked that the new system "is the first major change in the way physicians are paid since they stopped accepting chickens and pigs."

Since this book was first published in 1992, enormous changes have affected the health care industry: the advent of the prospective payment system; the spectacular growth of managed care as a payer; the explosion of health care systems;, and the formation of physician practice networks, physician companies, and other physician-owned entities. In 1992, health care was beginning to feel the early pressures of managed care and aggressive competition. Today, those pressures have shaken the health care industry (some would say for the better) to its foundations. Effective physician leadership is required throughout the health care industry.

Gains Since 1992

The number of physicians in MBA programs has increased significantly, as has the number of MBA programs for physician executives. The physician executive role within health systems is now better defined and more appropriately titled vice president for medical management. Managed care is here to stay, and new roles for medical executives are appearing daily. While the need for a physician executive was questioned in many organizations in 1992, in 1999 the need is more apparent than ever and the opportunities for physician executives are growing.

What the Future Holds

In the future, physician executives will be more firmly entrenched and needed in acute care settings, ambulatory settings, and all other businesses associated with a traditional hospital or hospital system. Physicians have and will continue to move into CEO roles in hospitals, health systems, and myriad health care-related organizations. Health care organizations are looking for physicians who can optimize revenue from clinical programs.

The alignment of health systems' business along service lines is rapidly accelerating. Service lines for cardiology, oncology, orthopedics, and women's health are becoming better defined as systems re-form in larger entities. The crossing of organizational lines with a continuum of services in each of these areas is not only apparent but necessary.

The implications for the work of physician-leadership search committees are easy to predict. In the short term, search committees will be charged with identifying candidates for clinical leadership roles who can help the hospital organization in its drastic shift from old, predictable relationships and in rebuilding revenue. Longer term clinical leaders who possess not only strong clinical skills but also management skills and leadership qualities will be needed. The difficulty may be finding leaders in a profession that trains its products to operate very independently and to work with relatively predictable outcomes. Leadership leans on team input and involvement and requires a risk on outcomes.

Managed care, while perceived as another "payer" in the past, is now a "player" on the health care scene. In addition to the traditional insurance-based managed care organization, medical executives from the "provider side" are sought by many managed care organizations. This will continue to be the case into the foreseeable future. Provider-owned HMOs and direct contracting by providers with employers will be the norm soon.

Physician practice networks, physician practice companies, physician/hospital equity organizations, and for-profit physician practice management companies are common today. New leadership will be needed in these organizations as they consolidate and become larger.

New opportunities in long-term care/continuing care services and behavioral health create additional venues for physician executives into the next millennium.

Academic medical centers will need new, decisive clinical/academic/executive leaders to survive. Chairs of clinical services with good business skills and management preparation will not come from within the traditional academic ranks. Recruitment of nonacademic chair/executives is already under way.

Kouzes and Posner observed that "those people who are most central to solving the organization's crucial problems and ensuring the company's long-term viability have the most power."* In today's environment of reduced revenue and increased competition, physician-leaders clearly are central to a health care organization's long-term viability and will clearly wield increasingly more power in the health care organization of the future.

---

*Kouzes, J., and Posner, B. *The Leadership Challenge: How to Get Extraordinary Things Done in Organizations*. San Francisco, Calif.: Jossey-Bass, 1990.

APPENDIX 1

ABC Hospital
Chairman, Obstetrics and Gynecology

SEARCH WORKPLAN

	April				May					June				July				August					September			
	5	12	19	26	3	10	17	24	31	7	14	21	28	5	12	19	26	2	9	16	23	31	6	13	20	27
Proposal Accepted	*																									
Information Gathering		—	—	—																						
Position Specification Submitted and Accepted					*																					
Candidate Identification			—	—	—	—	—	—	—	—	—	—														
Progress Report												*														
Candidate Interviews by L+S						—	—	—	—	—	—	—	—													
Client Interviews (1st Round)												—	—	—	—	—										
Client Interviews (2nd, 3rd round) Candidate															—	—	—	—	—	—						
Credentialing/Referencing																										
Candidate Offer/Acceptance															—	—	—	—	—				*			

APPENDIX 2

Sample Search Committee Structures

Setting:	Community Teaching Hospital 450 Beds
Position:	Chief of Oncology
Committee Size:	Ten members
Committee Chair:	Chief of Pathology

Members:

- Chief Operating Officer
- Chief of Radiation Oncology
- Chair of Medicine
- Director of Medical Education
- General Surgeon
- Oncologists (2 ex officio)
- Cardiologist
- Obstetrician/Gynecologist (2)
- Family Practitioner

Setting:	Medical College Hospital 300 Beds
Position:	Chairman of Surgery
Committee Size:	Eight members
Committee Chair:	Chairman of Pathology

Members:

- Professor, Physiology/Biochemistry (2)
- Assistant Professor, Obstetrics/Gynecology (gynecologic oncologist)
- Professor, Pathology
- Professor, Surgery
- Professor, Thoracic Surgery
- Clinical Professor, Department of Medicine
- Associate Professor, Emergency Medicine

Setting: Community Hospital
500 Beds

Position: Chief of Pathology
Committee Size: Eight members
Committee Chair: Vice President, Medical Affairs
Members:

- Urologist (also President of Medical Staff)
- Cardiologist
- Vice President, Professional Services
- Two Trustees

APPENDIX 3

Sample Pro Forma Income Statement: Hospital Pathology Services

($000s omitted)

Revenue:		
Professional Fees Collected[1]		$1,077
Part A Stipend[2]		298
	Net Revenue	$1,375
Expenses:		
Collection expense[3]		$118
Benefits[4]		159
Malpractice premiums		20
	Total Expenses	$297
Surplus (Loss)		$1,078

1. Market indicates a collection rate of between 60 and 80 percent of professional billings for pathology services. For purposes of this pro forma statement, we have assumed a collection rate of 70 percent of billings.
2. Supervision, teaching, administration, research.
3. Assumes the cost of an outside billing firm to be 11 percent of professional fees collected.
4. Assumes standard benefits to include health and life insurance, pension funding equal to 8 percent of compensation, short-term and long-term disability insurance, and legally mandated payroll deductions.

Source: L+S Pathology Market Study, 1991

APPENDIX 4

Minutes and Reports of Officers*

<u>Minutes:</u>

The record of the proceedings of a deliberative assembly is usually called the minutes, or sometimes—particularly in legislative bodies—the journal. In an ordinary society, unless the minutes are to be published, they should contain mainly a record of what was done at the meeting, not what was said by the members. The minutes should never reflect the secretary's opinion, favorable or otherwise, on anything said or done.

<u>Content of the Minutes:</u> The first paragraph of the minutes should contain the following information (which need not, however, be divided into numbered or separated items directly corresponding to those below):

1. the kind of meeting: regular, special, adjourned regular, or adjourned special;
2. the name of the society or assembly;
3. the date and time of the meeting, and the place, if it is not always the same;
4. the fact that the regular chair and secretary were present, or in their absence, the names of the persons who substituted for them; and
5. whether the minutes of the previous meeting were read and approved—as read, or as corrected—the date of that meeting being given if it was other than a regular business meeting.

The body of the minutes should contain a separate paragraph for each subject matter and should show:

6. all main motions or motions to bring a main question again before the assembly—except any that were withdrawn—giving:
   a. the wording in which each motion was adopted or otherwise disposed of (with the facts as to how the motion may have been debated or amended before disposition being mentioned only parenthetically);
   b. the disposition of the motion, including—if it was temporarily disposed of—any primary and secondary amendment and all adhering secondary motions that were then pending; and
   c usually, in the case of all important motions, the name of the mover;
7. all notices of motions; and
8. all points of order and appeals, whether sustained or lost, together with the reasons given by the chair for his ruling.

The last paragraph should state:

9. the hour of adjournment.

*Excerpted from *Robert's Rules of Order*, Glenview, Ill.: Scott Foresman and Company, 1970, pp. 389, 390.

APPENDIX 5

Draft Position Specification

<u>TITLE</u>

Physician-in-Chief, Division of Medical Oncology

<u>ORGANIZATION</u>

An accredited, acute care community teaching hospital located in a mid-Atlantic metropolitan area. This 450-bed regional medical center has an annual budget of $112 million and independent residency programs in Internal Medicine, Family Practice, General Surgery, and Obstetrics/Gynecology. It is an established leader in Oncology in its service area and wants to further develop its competitive presence in regional cancer care by becoming a designated Community Cancer Center. The institution's administration firmly believes that it has the "forces within" to compete and to do a superior job in the delivery of cancer care services. To this end, it has created a new Division of Oncology.

<u>RESPONSIBILITIES</u>

The successful physician candidate for this position will be an effective and charismatic leader with the vision and discretion to build consensus within the Division of Oncology. The new Physician-in-Chief will also play a key role in bringing a strong multidisciplinary team approach to community cancer care, inpatient care, and therapy. This individual will also have important responsibilities for educating primary care physicians with regard to both available skills within the Division and appropriate referral patterns.

The Physician-in-Chief, Division of Medical Oncology, should have the ability to lead the new Division and coordinate its interactions with other hospital departments and divisions, hospital administration, patients, and patient families. He or she will be a leader in the institution's efforts to project an image of superior cancer care that includes case-discovery outreach activities, design and implementation of treatment protocols, and support of the patient in the home environment, including planned and coordinated support for the family.

<u>REQUIREMENTS</u>

The candidate will have demonstrated leadership abilities, outstanding clinical skills, and a commitment to medical education. Additional requirements include but are not limited to the following:

- Demonstrated clinical expertise and recognition as a consultant physician, preferably in solid tumor oncology.
- An interest in developing community outreach programs and an appreciation of the role of hospice care in a far-sighted oncology program.
- Experience in clinical research and prior participation in oncology protocols (highly desirable).
- A minimum of 5 to 15 years of post-fellowship experience, to include significant administrative activity.

APPENDIX 6

Candidate Interview Agenda

Neal D. Conahan, MD
Candidate: Chairman, Cardiothoracic Surgery
Monday, June 21, 1999

7:30 a.m.	-	Barry Steinberg, President Alex Moran, FACHE, Vice President, Medical Staff Affairs and Patient Management Services Executive Offices
8:00 a.m.	-	Lawrence Alford, MD Catherine Sullivan, MD Members, Division of Cardiology Mathew Carson, MD, Acting Chief, Division of Cardiothoracic Surgery Founders Hall Conference Room Breakfast Meeting
9:00 a.m.	-	Danielle Hinton, Project Manager Tour
10:00 a.m.	-	Mack McDowd, Director, Perfusion Services Stephen Shore, Assistant Director, Perfusion Services Founders Hall Conference Room
11:00 a.m.	-	Susan Bellamy, MSN Clinical Director, Cardiovascular Nursing Founders Hall Conference Room
12:00 Noon	-	Muriel Alt Lunch and tour of residential areas
4:00 p.m.	-	Robert Doyle, MD Chief, Division of Cardiology Founders Hall Conference Room
5:00 p.m. 6:30 p.m.	-	Meeting with Search Committee Board Room

APPENDIX 7

ABC MEMORIAL HOSPITAL

Candidate Evaluation Form
Chairman, Department of Obstetrics and Gynecology

CANDIDATE: ____________________ SUBSPECIALTY: ________________

INSTITUTION: _________________ ACADEMIC RANK: _____________

	STRONG	ABOVE AVERAGE	AVERAGE	BELOW AVERAGE
LEADERSHIP STATURE • Vision • Initiatives • Accomplishments				
ADMINISTRATIVE EXPERIENCE • Scope of Responsibility • Management Ability • Contributions to medical center				
CLINICAL EXPERIENCE • Clinical Stature and Recognition • Area of Specialization • Clinical Program Development				
ACADEMIC STATURE • Society Membership/Posts • Quality of Publications • Regional/National Recognition				
TEACHING EXPERIENCE • Residents; Students; Fellows • Teaching and/or Recognition • Teaching Program Development				
INTERPERSONAL ABILITY • Sensitivity to Needs of General Staff • Communication Skills • Community Involvement and Interests				

CANDIDACY STATUS:	Briefly explain your choice:
____ FAVOR	
____ OPPOSE	
____ UNDECIDED	

Interview Date ________________

Search Committee Member Signature ________________

Source: L+S

APPENDIX 8

PHYSICIAN CREDENTIAL CHECK

(Education Through Certification)

CANDIDATE:

FACTOR		CONFIRMATION	
Undergraduate: City/State: Degree & Major: Date Bestowed:		Contact Name: Office: Telephone #: Date of Confirmation:	
Graduate: City/State: Degree & Major: Date Bestowed:		Contact: Office: Telephone #: Date of Confirmation:	
Medical School: City/State: Degree & Major: Date Bestowed:		Contact: Office: Telephone #: Date of Confirmation:	
Internship: Program: City/State: Dates in Program:		Contact Name: Office: Telephone #: Date of Confirmation:	
Residency: Program: City/State: Dates in Program:		Contact Name: Office: Telephone #: Date of Confirmation:	
LICENSURE			
State(s) Licensed in: License #: License Issued: Current Through: Status: Board Actions:		Contact Name: Office: Telephone: Date of Confirmation:	
Board Certification:		Verified By:	

PHYSICIAN CREDENTIAL CHECK

CANDIDATE:

EMPLOYMENT			
HOSPITAL		**CONFIRMATION**	
Employer:		Contact Name:	
City/State:		Office:	
Title/Rank:		Telephone #:	
Date Employed:		Date of Confirmation:	
Facility:		Contact Name:	
City/State:		Office:	
Title/Rank:		Telephone #:	
Date Employed:		Date of Confirmation:	
Facility:		Contact:	
City/State:		Office:	
Title/Rank:		Telephone #:	
Date Employed:		Date of Confirmation:	
Facility:		Contact Name:	
City/State:		Office:	
Title/Rank:		Telephone #:	
Dates Employed:		Date of Confirmation:	
ACADEMIC APPOINTMENT			
Facility:		Contact Name:	
City/State:		Office:	
Title/Rank:		Telephone #:	
Dates Employed:		Date of Confirmation:	
Facility:		Contact Name:	
City/State:		Office:	
Title/Rank:		Telephone #:	
Dates Employed:		Date of Confirmation:	

APPENDIX 9

Sample Reference Reports

REFERENCE:	James. L. McGinn, MD
CANDIDATE FOR:	Chairman, Department of Medicine Program Director, Internal Medicine Residency

---

GIVEN BY:	James Hamilton, MD, MPH Private Practice Physician Wilmington, Delaware
DATE:	July 9, 1998

Dr. Hamilton has known Dr. McGinn since 1982 when Dr. Hamilton was a resident at the University of Wilmington. He has interacted with Dr. McGinn on a resident/teacher basis as well as a collegial basis. Dr. Hamilton had the following comments concerning Dr. McGinn:

- "I would describe Jim McGinn as a first-rate person, someone with a lot of talent in a lot of areas. His clinical skills are superb and he is in my mind a natural-born leader. Jim is a guy who is very entrepreneurial, with a sense of vision and commitment to his specialty."
- "Jim's teaching skills are exemplary and he is an outstanding role model for residents and fellows. I know that all the people that I trained with thought very highly of him and sought him out for his opinions."
- "I think any community teaching hospital is lucky to get someone like Jim McGinn. He has accomplished quite a lot at University Medical Center in such a short period of time, and for anyone with a strong clinical orientation to succeed as quickly as he has at an academic center such as University Medical Center is unusual and certainly speaks to his credit. I know that he is an Associate Dean for the medical school and is also being considered for Chief of the Medical Staff. University Medical Center certainly thinks highly of Jim McGinn and I think that is a pretty good reference in and of itself."
- "Jim has the ability to lead a Department of Medicine at a community teaching hospital such as Memorial. Jim has been a private practitioner himself; he knows the day-to-day realities in running one's own practice and he knows how to get voluntary staff involved in the teaching programs. Just look at what he has done at University Medical Center. He has built a very solid, well-respected fellowship program in rheumatology there and he has done that by getting the voluntary staff and the full-time faculty to work together."

- "When Jim was here at the University of Wilmington, he served as a member of the Public Health Council for the State of Delaware. This is a seven-member committee with two of the members being physicians. This is a very political body which allocates money for capital projects in the State of Delaware. Jim was appointed to the council by the governor. I think it is certainly to Jim's credit that he was chosen to serve on such a committee. It certainly speaks to his outstanding reputation and his leadership potential."

- "There is no area in which I think Jim needs any improvement. I have always found him to be an impressive individual, hard working and very astute. I don't mean to sound flippant but your community hospital should really jump at the chance to have a Jim McGinn as its Chairman of Medicine."

REFERENCE:	James. L. McGinn, MD
CANDIDATE FOR:	Chairman, Department of Medicine Program Director, Internal Residency
GIVEN BY:	Samuel Mayson, MD Professor, Radiology and Cell Biology University of Wilmington Wilmington, Delaware
DATE:	July 14, 1998

Dr. Mayson has been a faculty member at the University of Wilmington for most of his career. He taught Dr. McGinn when Dr. McGinn was a medical student here and frequently interacted with him when Dr. McGinn returned to the university in 1979 as a research associate. Dr. Mayson had the following comments concerning Dr. McGinn:

- "I've known Dr. McGinn since he was a medical student here at the University of Wilmington. Throughout the years, while Dr. McGinn was a medical student and when he joined the faculty here, we have worked on several research projects together and have collaborated on several publications. Without hesitation, I can absolutely recommend Dr. McGinn for the Chairman of Medicine position at Memorial Hospital. I have seen Dr. McGinn in clinical, research, and teaching situations, and he has always performed outstandingly."

- "Jim McGinn has excellent leadership abilities. I saw those abilities at work here at the University of Wilmington in his handling of residents and fellows and in his professional interactions with other members of the staff. He is a good communicator who is highly respected and whose opinions are sought after."

- "Jim is well-known within his specialty and is well-respected. He is an excellent clinician who has made a name for himself in rheumatology. I don't think he could have accomplished what he did out at University Medical Center without such a reputation."

- "Jim is a good idea man and knows how to put his ideas into play. I would also describe him as a people person, someone who can motivate and get people working together. He is most definitely a team player and not one to make unilateral decisions."

- "While here at the University of Wilmington, he got on quite well with the faculty and the voluntary staff. I think if you talk with other faculty members here or to the private practice physicians you won't find anyone who did not like him or respect him."

- "Jim has an entrepreneurial bent which manifested itself in the development of his own private practice while he was here at the University of Wilmington. He built up this practice on his own initiative without assistance from the university. He has taken those same skills and has applied them to his position at University Medical Center. He is a person who can get things done in a short period of time."

- "The only area where I think he can use a bit of improvement is in trimming down his agenda. He takes on a lot of activities, and quite frankly I don't know how he gets it all done but he does. I think he may at times allow himself to get pulled in too many directions at once. There are some people, though, who would not consider this a failing. But regardless, Memorial will be getting a high-energy individual who has impeccable clinical skills, solid leadership ability and is one of the best academic physicians that you will find. I don't think that your hospital can do any better."

APPENDIX 10

Sample Matrix: Chairman of Anesthesia

	Candidate A	Candidate B	Candidate C
EXPERIENCE	Since 7/86, Staff Anesthesiologist & Director of Critical Care at large teaching hospital in Philadelphia Area. Additional five years post fellowship experience as Director ICU & Asst. Professor of Anesthesia, Medicine & Surgery at large Level 1 trauma center in New York.	Chairman, Dept. of Anesthesia for past 10 years at 250+bed community hospital in Pennsylvania. Prior experience includes staff responsibilities at same hospital.	Since 1983, independent anesthesiologist at 400+bed teaching affiliate of university medical school in New England.
Administrative Responsibilities	Significant	Significant	Moderate
EDUCATION			
M.D. Degree	University of Pittsburgh (1970)	University of Pennsylvania (1972)	Chicago Medical School (1980)
Anesthesiology Residency	HUP, Philadelphia, PA (1984 - 1986) (Earlier had residencies in IM)	HUP Philadelphia, PA (1973 - 1975)	Columbia Presbyterian Medical Center New York, NY (1981 - 1983)
Fellowship	Pulmonary Diseases Duke University (1971 - 1972) Baylor College of Medicine (1977 - 1978)	Anesthesiology HUP/Philadelphia, PA (1975 - 1976)	None
ACADEMIC APPOINTMENT	Yes	None Current	Yes
LICENSURE	Pennsylvania	Pennsylvania	New Jersey
CERTIFICATION	IM; PD; Anesthesiology; CC	Anesthesiology	Anesthesiology
COMPENSATION	$185K (Salary)	$200K (FFS)	$225 (FFS)

	Candidate D	Candidate E	Candidate F
EXPERIENCE	Since 1976, partner in anesthesiology group providing services to 900+bed teaching hospital system & community hospital in northern New York. For five years had overlapping responsibility as Director of Education/Department of Anesthesia.	Since 1986, Co-Director of Department of Anesthesia at 300+bed community hospital in North Carolina. Prior experience includes two years at TJUH and three years as Staff/Director at a community hospital in Pennsylvania.	Following five years as Assistant Chairman, promoted to Chairman in 1984 of a 500+bed hospital in western Pennsylvania.
Administrative Responsibilities	Significant	Significant	Significant
EDUCATION			
M.D. Degree	University of Pennsylvania (1973)	Bowman Gray - North Carolina (1974)	SUNY - Buffalo (1969)
Anesthesiology Residency	HUP Philadelphia, PA (1974 - 1976)	HUP Philadelphia, PA (1975 - 1977)	Albert Einstein College of Medicine New York, NY (1970 - 1972)
Fellowship	None	Cardiac and Neuro-Anesthesia	CT Anesthesia Albert Einstein College of Medicine, NY (1972 - 1973)
ACADEMIC APPOINTMENT	None Current	Yes	Yes
LICENSURE	Pennsylvania, New York	North Carolina, Pennsylvania	Pennsylvania
CERTIFICATION	Anesthesiology	Anesthesiology	Anesthesiology
COMPENSATION	$230K (FFS)	$250K+ (FFS) estimated	$300K+ (FFS)

APPENDIX 11

Physician Leadership Compensation Ranges

Position	Compensation Range
Chairperson, Anesthesia	$215,000 - $500,000
Chairperson, Cardiology	$175,000 - $350,000
Chairperson, Emergency Medicine	$175,000 - $325,000
Chairperson, Medicine	$220,000 - $300,000
Chairperson, Obstetrics and Gynecology	$250,000 - $350,000
Chairperson, Pathology	$225,000 - $375,000
Chairperson, Pediatrics	$225,000 - $375,000
Chairperson, Physiatry	$200,000 - $400,000
Chairperson, Radiation Oncology	$250,000 - $800,000
Chairperson, Radiology	$200,000 - $280,000
Chairperson, Surgery	$275,000 - $475,000
Chief, CT Surgery	$250,000 - $1,000,000
Director, Infectious Disease	$130,000 - $300,000
Director, Neonatology	$150,000 - $300,000
Director, Nephrology	$140,000 - $200,000
Director, Oncology Program	$175,000 - $300,000
Program Director, Family Practice	$150,000 - $200,000
Program Director, Medicine	$150,000 - $175,000

APPENDIX 12

Anesthesia Department
Analysis of Clinical Income

Revenue Estimate Assumptions

- Revenue = (Base Units + Time Units) x Conversion Factor
- Unit charge rate = $45.00
- Average time = 90 minutes/15 minutes = 6 time units
- Average base units = 5 base units

Total Units = 11 units

- Total cases = 4,800 x 11 units = 52,800 total units

Breakdown by payer		Units
– Medicare	60%	
Personally 20%		6,336
Supervised 80%		25,344
– HMO	12%	6,336
– Blue Shield	11%	5,808
– Commercial	10%	5,280
– Self-Pay	4%	2,112
– Medicaid	3%	1,584
Total	100%	52,800

Anesthesia Department
Revenue Calculation

	Units	Reimbursement Per Unit	Revenue
Medicare - M.D. Revenue			
Personally Performed	6,336	$17.24	$109,233
Supervised[a]	12,672[a]	$17.24	218,465
Sub Total			$327,698
Medicare - CRNA Revenue[a]	12,672[a]	$17.24	$218,465
HMO	6,336	$13.14	$ 83,255
Blue Shield	5,808	$21.00	$121,968
Commercial	5,280	$28.00	$147,840
Self Pay	2,112	$ 3.50	$ 7,392
Medicaid	1,584	$ 8.75	$ 13,860
Total	52,800 units		$920,478

Note: [a]Medicare supervised units at 50% for anesthesiologist and CRNA.

APPENDIX 13

Sample Letter of Intent

(date)

Dear Doctor:

The Medical and Administrative Staff you have met during your two visits to ABC Hospital are enthusiastic about the prospects of recruiting you to ABC Hospital. This letter is intended to restate and to formalize the preliminary offer that I made to you by telephone last Friday evening.

ABC Hospital proposes that you be employed by XYZ Professional Services Corporation (a not-for-profit entity providing specialty physician services to our area) under the following terms.

A. Initial contract term of two years, with provisions for renewal on an annual basis thereafter (evergreen provision).

B. Annual base compensation for the first year of $195,000, increasing to $210,000 for the second year, and $225,000 for the third year.

C. Parity with Drs. Smith and Jones beginning the fourth year of the arrangement.

D. A provision commencing in the fourth year providing for additional compensation if the activity of the practice exceeds predefined levels.

E. Benefit package that includes health insurance (family plan), dental insurance, life insurance, disability insurance, pension plan, FICA.

F. Malpractice insurance.

G. Office space, office support staff, and billing services (to be provided through an arrangement with Professional Billing Associates).

H. Reimbursement of up to $5,000 for the services of a professional moving company.

As we discussed, this offer is contingent upon the outcome of a physician examination (which is required of all new physician employees), successful completion of the credentialing process at ABC Hospital, and approval of the arrangement by the Hospital's Board of Trustees.

If this proposal is acceptable to you, I suggest the next step is to schedule you for another visit where we can review contractual documents and discuss the arrangements in greater detail with both Drs. Smith and Jones, and with myself. You may also want to look at housing during this visit.

I look forward to hearing from you at your earliest convenience.

Sincerely,

Chief Executive Officer